First Aid for Horse and Rider

✚

Presented by *Colorado Country Life* magazine
and your local Electric Cooperative.

First Aid for Horse and Rider

Emergency Care for the Stable and Trail

Nancy S. Loving, DVM

and Gilbert Preston, MD

THE LYONS PRESS
Guilford, Connecticut
An imprint of The Globe Pequot Press

To buy books in quantity for corporate use
or incentives, call **(800) 962–0973**
or e-mail **premiums@GlobePequot.com.**

The Lyons Press is an imprint of The Globe Pequot Press

Illustrations by Teal Blake

Text design by Sheryl P. Kober

Library of Congress Cataloging-in-Publication Data is available on file.

ISBN 978-1-59921-293-7

Printed in the United States of America

10 9 8 7 6 5 4 3 2 1

CAUTION
Outdoor recreational activities are by their nature potentially hazardous. In all cases, the first aid measures in this book are meant only as suggestions for general situations and cannot cover all first aid crises that might occur. Proper medical evaluation of each individual or horse is necessary to accurately diagnose and treat a problem. The authors are not responsible for decisions made or medical care rendered by an individual to another individual or horse when professional medical advice is not obtained. The goal of this book is to help you reach professional medical care safely and in reasonable comfort, and none of the advice given here is intended to replace professional care whenever it is available.

Contents

Part One: The Horse by Nancy S. Loving, DVM

Contents

{Nancy S. Loving, DVM}

Introduction

Within these pages on first aid care of the horse, the objective is to give you, the owner, various tools to identify what might be a true emergency and how to handle an emergency while awaiting professional veterinary expertise. Although not every circumstance can be addressed within this book, you can read about common emergency situations that you are likely to encounter with a horse, whether riding in the wilderness or at the barn. Each topic provides practical methods to give you a starting place to handle the situation. Being armed with basic information will provide you with a degree of calm when faced with a crisis and allow you to be effective in dealing with the problem.

The veterinary medical suggestions in this section are meant for horses only and are not meant for application to human problems. In all cases, described veterinary first aid measures are only meant as suggestions for a general situation, and they cannot cover all first aid crises or specific idiosyncrasies that might occur. Not all horses are amenable to handling and treatment when in pain, so don't assume that a horse will always be receptive to your efforts.

Once the immediate crisis has been addressed, seek professional veterinary advice and expertise to ensure the best possible care for your horse. Have your horse evaluated as soon as possible by a veterinarian who can accurately diagnose and treat the problem. In no way should the information or suggestions within this book be construed to provide a diagnosis or a cure, but rather should be used as guidelines to improve a horse's comfort and to minimize the consequences of an immediate crisis.

For detailed horse health care information, please refer to my comprehensive book, *All Horse Systems Go: The Horse Owner's Full-Color Veterinary Care and Conditioning Resource for Modern Performance, Sport and Pleasure Horses.*

Best of luck!

Nancy S. Loving, DVM
July 2007

2.

Medical History and Action Plans

Whether you are off enjoying yourself on a wilderness riding or camping expedition, on your way to or attending a horse show or event, or simply at the farm or the barn preparing to ride or care for your horse, there are times when an equine emergency arises, necessitating rapid but sensible decisions. Being prepared in advance is invaluable.

Medical Details about Your Horse

Some horses have specific medical problems or behavioral quirks that should be disclosed to others assisting you and your horse, or to a veterinarian rendering medical care. It is helpful to provide written details on a laminated card that is carried in proximity to the horse, or placed on his stall or enclosure in the event that you cannot be contacted. In appropriate situations, put all written instructions in both English and Spanish so these are understood by all barn personnel.

Examples of relevant information include:

- Known allergies, particularly to specific medications and foods. Mark these in bold and in red.

- Behavioral quirks that make the horse dangerous to handle, such as tendencies to strike, kick, run over you, bite, or explode.

- Incompatibilities with certain horses or with any living arrangements.

- Specific dietary requirements or restrictions.

Action Plan for When You Are Not Available

Not all emergency events with horses occur when you are around, so it is best to be proactive in your planning. You may be out of town or unavailable when your horse experiences an emergency crisis, so it is important to leave the following in writing with responsible agents caring for the horse:

- Your contact information.

- Name and contact information for the insurance company, which must be notified prior to any medical procedures (if the horse is insured).

- Name and contact information for person(s) willing to act as a decision-making agent on your behalf.

- List of veterinarians you authorize to tend to your horse and contact numbers.

- Specific allergies your horse may have, especially to medication.

- How much money you are willing to spend on emergency medical and/or surgical treatment if someone is unable to contact you in a timely fashion.

- Arrangements for transport of horse to hospital or surgical facility if this becomes necessary.

- List of persons willing to transport your horse in your absence.

- Whether you are willing to authorize emergency surgery, if necessary.

- Authorization of euthanasia if that is the only humane option for your horse.
- Current credit card information provided to your agent and/or veterinarian.

When You Are Present During an Emergency

Keeping a calm mind when faced with an emergency sometimes takes practice, while some people are gifted with a cool demeanor during a crisis. To best prepare for an emergency so you can respond appropriately and in a timely fashion, it is helpful to have already done the following:

- Know how your horse behaves during normal times so you can recognize when something is wrong (see Assessing Vital Signs, page 10).
- Have all first aid materials and supplies on hand in an easily accessible area (see First Aid Kit, page 100).
- Familiarize yourself with layman's terms for your horse's body parts, particularly the legs, so you can communicate these accurately to your veterinarian.
- Read through this book in advance to familiarize yourself with where to locate certain topics and to give you an idea of what could go wrong and what might be an appropriate response.

3.

When Both the Horse and Rider Are Injured

There are occasions when a horse and rider suffer a mishap together, such as stepping in a hole or a bog, getting caught in a landslide, falling over the side of a cliff, or another disaster. Sometimes the rider is thrown and the spooked horse runs off and gets injured. If a rider is injured so severely that she or he is unable to catch the horse or find a way to get help, then that goes beyond the scope of the topics of first aid covered in this book; each such situation must be handled individually. This book is a general resource and not meant as specific medical advice for your exact situation, especially since it is not possible to anticipate all potential scenarios you might encounter. It might be wise to contact your physician in advance and discuss possible options should you find yourself badly injured in the wilderness. Also, please refer to Part II: The Rider, in this book.

I can make some suggestions that are based on my personal experiences with injury. I live in an area that abuts a national forest, providing me with ample opportunities to ride alone in the wilderness. These suggestions are ideas that I've formulated to provide myself protection from serious mishap over the past thirty-five years of trail riding and do not apply to all situations, riders, or horses. Hopefully some of these suggestions will prove useful to you. You may have other practical ideas to share with your friends, as well.

Proactive Preventive Strategies

Always leave information at your barn or with someone at home as to where you will be riding, especially if venturing out alone. Do not deviate from this plan no matter how interesting another trail may look once you start your ride. If you leave your intended route, then no one will know where to look for you should you get lost or injured.

Also, provide information about what time you will leave the barn or trailer and how long you plan to be gone. This will enable people to determine if you are overdue for your anticipated return.

Have your cell phone on your person with a fully charged battery (along with a spare battery). A phone may not work in all areas you may ride, but if you are with someone else or help arrives, that person can ride or drive to an area that has cell service.

Ride with one or more capable people whenever possible. This is particularly important if your horse is not entirely trustworthy.

Check the weather forecast in advance and be sure you are prepared for rapid weather changes.

Carry a first aid kit in a cantle pack that provides emergency supplies for both you and your horse.

Have emergency supplies (and essential personal medications) with you on your person in an accessible place in case you become separated from your horse. (See below for a list of essential items)

To Catch a Loose Horse

If you are thrown from your horse and you or a friend is able to attempt to catch him, usually the bridle and reins are still attached. But if, for some reason, your horse has lost his head restraint, you can put your belt around his neck as a temporary halter. It is a good idea to travel with an extra halter or long rope in your saddle bag in the event that a bridle or reins break. If you elect to ride with a rope halter beneath your horse's bridle, be sure it is made of material that will break if you get separated and the horse runs loose. Otherwise, he could snag it on a protrusion (or his foot when scratching) and cause himself serious injury.

If the horse is panicked or tangled in tack or equipment, care must be taken not to put yourself in harm's way. Look around the area and make sure you won't be trapped against an obstacle or along a waterway or ditch when approaching the horse. Leave yourself plenty of room to maneuver and to get away quickly.

Generally, a horse will remain in the vicinity of other horses, so if you wait for the panicked horse to calm down, he may stop in his tracks and rest for a bit before attempting to explode again. Have a sharp pocketknife handy to cut him free from entanglements when possible. Each situation will be different, but common sense should prevail. Do not put yourself in harm's way.

To Free a Trapped Horse

There are occasions when a horse falls off a precipice, gets trapped in a bog, or is stuck in a ditch. There is no way for you to forcibly remove the horse from such a situation, and you will need to obtain professional help from a rescue crew well versed in these types of crises. Attempt to calm the horse when possible, and call for help.

A trapped or injured horse will be reacting on instinct and may be thrashing to free himself or to get up. Remember that he is still a large, powerful animal, and if in pain or trapped, he can be extremely unpredictable. Even the most well-trained, level-headed horses can turn into frightened, dangerous creatures. Try to get clear of his space to protect yourself from being hurt by him.

Essential Items to Carry on Your Person

Some horses will run off if you are thrown, while on other occasions you might be so injured that you cannot rise from the ground. There are a few items that could make the difference if you carry them on your person. If you have concerns about getting separated from your horse, it is best to wear a small waist pack carried in front, with the contents over your belly rather than your back. If you were to land on your back, a protruding pack could cause injury to your spine or pelvis. A fishing vest is a handy place to secure items and have them remain accessible. Try to shield hard materials within softer ones in case you are thrown.

Items to include in your personal waist pack or vest:

- Cell phone with fully charged battery.
- List of pertinent phone numbers to contact help.
- Personal medications.
- Health insurance card and information.
- Matches in a waterproof container.
- Small "survival" or "space" blanket (A thin sheet of waterproof and windproof material that is coated with a metallic reflective agent that reflects body heat back to the body.)
- Light windbreaker or waterproof jacket.
- Energy bar(s).
- Full flask of water.
- Pocket knife.
- Flare.

4.

Assessing Vital Signs

Record all findings of a horse's vital signs, documenting the time the information was obtained and the results. This allows you to track progress or deterioration of the horse's condition.

Heart Rate

Using a stethoscope (inexpensive ones are available through catalogs or at a pharmacy) count the number of beats per minute (bpm) by placing the end of the stethoscope on the body wall just behind and at the level of the left elbow. Each *lub-dub* you hear counts as one beat.

- The normal resting heart rate for a horse is 28 to 40 bpm.

- Pain will often drive a horse's heart rate up to 64 bpm.

- Critical problems like shock or an intestinal twist will cause a horse's heart rate to rise over 80 bpm, and it will remain elevated. Sometimes a spasm of pain will cause transient elevation, so check the heart rate again in ten to fifteen minutes.

- Rapid breathing, obvious signs of pain and distress, or depression often accompany a rapid heart rate.

Respiratory Rate

Count the number of respirations per minute. You can do this by counting each diaphragm lift visible in the flank area. Or, hold your hand in front of the horse's nostrils and count each breath.

The number of respirations per minute gives an indication of whether the horse is normal or stressed:

- Normal respiratory rate in a resting horse is twelve to twenty-four breaths per minute.

- Arduous exercise, or overheating from fever or heat stress, will cause an elevation in the respiratory rate.

- High ambient temperatures, particularly with high humidity, may elicit a rapid respiratory rate in the absence of any problem.

- A horse that is panting has a high respiratory rate, often at a count faster than the heart rate; this is called an inversion.

Mucous Membranes

Lift the upper lip of your horse's mouth and look at the gum color above the teeth. Or, look beneath the upper eyelid, or just inside the lips of a mare's vulva.

- Membranes should be pink and moist, like the pink color you see beneath your fingernails.

- Pale pink color indicates decreased circulation, anemia, blood loss, or systemic illness.

- Bright red membranes indicate moderate stages of shock.

- Muddy-looking membranes indicate poor circulation, usually due to advanced shock.

- Yellow-hued membranes are often associated with liver stagnation, or may have little clinical significance other than indicating the horse has been eating legume plants.

Capillary Refill Time

Blanch the membranes of your horse's upper gum by pressing it with the tip of your finger, and note how quickly the pink color returns.

- Normal capillary refill time (CRT) should return the gums to a pink color in less than two seconds.

- Delayed CRT indicates cardiovascular compromise, often associated with dehydration or acute blood loss. (See Dehydration or Shock, page 33.)

Intestinal Sounds

With your stethoscope, listen to both sides of the flank for sounds similar to what you'd hear when your stomach rumbles when you're hungry.

- Over a couple of minutes, you should hear at least two or three intestinal rumbles in each quadrant of the flanks.

- A hyperactive gut may be noisy due to gaseous activity from over-fermenting feedstuffs or may be an early effort to move an impaction; loud sounds may precede complete intestinal shutdown.

- Occasional noises that sound similar to that of a penny

falling down a well (*tink-tink-tink-tink-tink*) may be heard on the right side of the flanks. This indicates gas in the cecum and intestinal stagnation.

• Absolute quiet is worrisome, as that indicates an absence of intestinal motility with increased risk of intestinal displacement or torsion.

Rectal Temperature

A rectal thermometer can be of any size or type (regular or digital) but the large animal type (which is five inches long) works best. Attach a string with some kind of clip (such as an alligator clip) to hook onto the horse's tail so you don't have to hold it with your fingers.

First, shake down the thermometer to a temperature that reads less than 96 degrees Fahrenheit. Then, lubricate the thermometer with petroleum jelly, ointment, or spit. To insert the thermometer, face backwards and stand to the side of the horse's hip, and only continue if the horse tolerates thermometer insertion into the rectum. If he tries to kick, it may not be safe to proceed. Leave the thermometer in place for about two minutes.

Read the temperature to see if your horse is within normal range or has a fever:

• Normal temperature for an adult horse is anything less than 101ºF.

• Normal temperature for a foal is considered anything less than 102ºF.

Any reading above these temperatures in a resting horse is considered a fever, particularly if there are other clinical signs, like depression or depressed appetite.

An exercising horse may have an elevated rectal temperature, which should decline steadily to a normal range over a twenty-minute period once exercise has stopped. An exercising horse typically works within a rectal temperature range of 101 to 103ºF. If rectal temperature surpasses 103.5ºF, the horse is overheating. (See Heat Stress, page 36.)

Hydration

A rider can determine a rough estimate of a horse's hydration. Grab a fold of skin on the point of the shoulder or an upper eyelid, and note how quickly it snaps back into position. Normally, the skin snaps back immediately.

- Skin that remains tented and refuses to return to its normal position may represent serious, life-threatening dehydration of 7 to 10 percent. This determination should be corroborated with other clinical parameters. There are many dehydration levels in between.

- A horse with mild dehydration (2 to 3 percent) also has a relatively dry mouth and dry mucous membranes.

- At about 5 percent dehydration, the eye sockets appear sunken in, skin elasticity is markedly reduced, the mucous membranes are tacky, and the horse is weak with a dull or listless attitude and posture.

Presence and Level of Pain

One additional vital sign to assess is that of pain. Is it present, and to what degree? Pain can be due to a variety of abdominal (intestinal), musculoskeletal, or thoracic (related to the lungs or the heart) causes:

- A horse with mild abdominal pain may be depressed or off feed, showing occasional and intermittent signs as seen with moderate pain (see Colic, page 19).

- A horse with moderate abdominal pain may be depressed, be off feed, paw the ground, roll the upper lip (flehmen), bite at his flanks, kick at his belly, lie down for unusually long periods, or occasionally roll on the ground (see Colic, page 19).

- A horse with severe abdominal pain may thrash around, get up and down unable to find a comfortable position to rest, roll violently on the ground, grind his teeth, hold his face in a grimace, and be unmanageable to control due to pain (see Colic, page 19).

- A horse with mild musculoskeletal pain may demonstrate poor performance, or may limp, or hold a leg or stand in an awkward position, or he may shift his weight from limb to limb (see Acute Lameness, page 76).

- A horse with moderate musculoskeletal pain will show a demonstrable limp, be reluctant to fully weight the painful leg, may walk in exaggerated fashion in attempts to relieve pressure on the sore area, or may bite at the bothersome leg (see Acute Lameness, page 76).

- A horse with severe musculoskeletal pain may be non-weight-bearing, or may act depressed or colicky (see Colic, page 19; see Acute Lameness, page 76).

- A horse with thoracic pain, related to injury, inflammation or infection of the lungs, ribs, or other chest anatomy, may be depressed, off feed, and/or may behave as with varying degrees of intestinal pain as described above.

5.

Intestinal Upset

Anytime you see a change in the amount or consistency of your horse's manure, you should be on the lookout for a reason. During times when your horse is passing normal feces, take note of how many piles of manure he produces over a twenty-four-hour period; this enables you to recognize when quantity is decreased. Also get an impression of the consistency and size of fecal balls he passes under normal conditions.

Diarrhea

If your horse has diarrhea:

- Gather vital signs (see Assessing Vital Signs, page 10).

- Monitor your horse to see if there are any obvious signs of discomfort (see Colic, page 19).

- Check if there is any malodor to the feces.

- Is the manure formed at all, or is it just runny or squirting watery feces? If formed somewhat, then you may be able to monitor for a bit without deeming this a true emergency. If the horse is passing squirting, watery feces, then you'll need to contact a veterinarian. If the horse is acting sick, call immediately. Otherwise, you should contact your vet as soon as possible during regular office hours.

FIRST STEPS

- Clean up all areas of diarrhea in the stall and paddock and on the horse's rump so you can determine when diarrhea clears up.

- If on grass, remove the horse from pasture and put in a dry lot or stall.

- Eliminate all grain products and supplements from the diet, offering only grass hay.

- Administer 4 ounces of bismuth subsalicylate every four hours by oral dose syringe. You can do this for two to three days, but if diarrhea is not resolving, stop medicating and contact your vet.

- Administer psyllium (at manufacturer's recommended dose) in a small amount of complete feed pellets. Repeat daily for several days to a week, provided the horse continues to improve.

- Provide free choice salt, and if the horse is drinking, then add one ounce of salt to each meal (mix it into as small an amount of pelleted feed or mashed beet pulp as possible) if the horse will eat it.

- If diarrhea does not improve within twenty-four to forty-eight hours, contact your veterinarian.

Scant or No Manure

If your horse is producing little or no manure, there is concern that he may be brewing an impaction that could progress to colic signs.

- Gather vital signs (see Assessing Vital Signs, page 10).

- Monitor water intake and urinary output.

- Confine the horse to a clean paddock or stall that allows you to monitor manure output.

- If any manure is present, look for signs of intestinal stagnation, such as mucous-coated feces (a gelatinous, light-colored material that coats the manure).

- If output does not improve within six to twelve hours, then contact your veterinarian immediately.

- Contact a veterinarian immediately if the horse is colicky or has not passed manure for six to twelve hours.

6.

Colic

Regardless of where you are or what you are doing, a horse is able to develop a bellyache, also called colic. Colic may be due to gas or spasms, while other colic events are more serious and caused by an impaction, intestinal displacement, or a twisted loop of bowel (torsion).

Signs of Colic Pain

A horse with colic can show a variety of clinical signs (see Fig. 1):
- Depression

- Absent or decreased appetite.

- Looking at one or both flanks while acting as if very uncomfortable.

- Flehmen (rolling up the upper lip).

- Pawing.

- Kicking at the belly.

- Lying down.

- Rolling on the ground.

- Anxious or distressed behavior.

What Should You Do?

Besides remaining calm, what should you do?

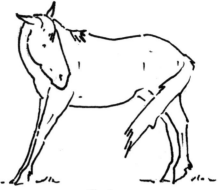

Fig. 1

First, determine how serious your horse's bellyache may be.

- Gather information about your horse's vital signs (see Assessing Vital Signs, page 10). Note that early stages of a serious colic may not yet elicit high heart rates or dramatic pain.

- Encourage the horse to get to his feet and see if he'll stand quietly.

- If he remains uncomfortable, put him on a longe line or in an arena and work him at a vigorous trot for about ten minutes. Sometimes this trotting motion dissipates gas to relieve a simple colic.

- If, following this bit of exercise, he still hasn't improved and shows no interest in food, it is time to call for veterinary help.

A horse that won't get up is often in significant pain, possibly but not necessarily due to colic. Something bothers him enough that he is oblivious to your urgings, or you aren't trying hard enough. You may need to smack the horse firmly and repeatedly (but humanely) on the haunches to stimulate him to rise, or you can try closing off his breathing by squeezing his nostrils shut for less than a minute. This usually will stimulate him to rise.

After trying the trot technique, if your horse remains uncomfortable or without appetite, and if he lies down again, but will rest quietly, then leave him be. He is better off conserving his energy resources by resting calmly either on his feet or prone on the ground. But if he tries to thrash or roll violently, it may be better to walk him to keep him from injuring himself. Be sure to protect yourself from getting in a position where you could be trapped or injured if he becomes violently painful.

Medicating a colicking horse with non-steroidal anti-inflammatory drugs, such as flunixin meglumine (Banamine®) or phenylbutazone paste (bute), without first conferring with your vet can be fraught with problems, like increasing the risk of developing gastric ulcers or kidney failure. But of significant consequence, these drugs can mask signs of a condition that requires immediate surgical intervention.

Colic Related to Non-Intestinal Problems

Other issues may cause a horse to act like he has colic when in fact his intestines are just fine. Some examples might be the horse that is tying up (myositis), a mare beginning labor for foaling, a horse with pleuropneumonia, a horse that is choking on feed, or a horse with painful laminitis.

- First, see if a recumbent horse will rise from the ground.

- Then, gather all the vital signs to try to differentiate what is going on (see Assessing Vital Signs, page 10).

7.

Choke

A "choking" horse is an emergency that arises while the horse is eating. Choke refers to an obstruction in the horse's esophagus, unlike in people, who choke due to an airway obstruction. (Although the anatomy of the esophagus and larynx is similar in function for people and horses, horses don't get food lodged in their airway as do people, but rather food becomes lodged in the horse's esophagus after it has been swallowed.) Choke is most likely to happen if a horse is fed pellets or horse cookies or similar dry and coarse material, and may occur in the horse trailer on the way to or from a riding spot. If you are camping in the wilderness, current requirements dictate that you use certified weed-free hay or certified pelleted feed to which your horse may be unaccustomed. Then the risk of choke is increased, especially if your horse is slightly dehydrated and not producing sufficient saliva in his mouth, or if he bolts this new and interesting feed without properly chewing it before swallowing.

Clinical Signs of Choke

- Mucus mixed with green frothy material is usually seen exiting the nose, as food material and mucus back up behind an obstruction in the esophagus. (see Fig. 2).

- A choked horse gags and coughs repeatedly in an effort to relieve the blockage.

- He may act colicky or distressed, and may even throw himself on the ground.

First Steps

You can try a few things before hauling the horse to veterinary help.

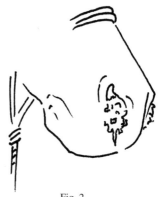

Fig. 2

- Place the horse on an incline with his head pointing down the hill. One danger of choke is aspiration pneumonia that develops because the horse inhales material as he coughs and gags in attempts to relieve the obstruction in his esophagus. The head-down position slightly minimizes the risk of inhaling food, saliva, and mucus.

- If available and with veterinary advisement, administer a short-acting intramuscular sedative or oxytocin to relieve spasms associated with the obstruction. The sedative also relaxes the horse's head and neck into a downward and extended position. Ideally, a choke might relieve itself if the horse relaxes.

- Withhold food and water until you are sure a choke is entirely resolved.

Prevention

Prevention is always the best cure. Either refrain from using pelleted feed, place large rocks in the feed bucket to slow your horse's intake, or mix the pellets into a gruel or mash by pre-soaking with water before feeding.

8.

Grain Overload

Even the most diligent horse owner can encounter the scenario of a horse loose on the premises, with free access to grain and rich feed. If you see piles of manure scattered around where they shouldn't be, it is likely that your horse has been rummaging around the vicinity for quite some time. A carbohydrate (grain) overload is a life-threatening condition because it can induce crippling laminitis in the hooves, create endotoxemia, cause colic, or cause the stomach to rupture due to the highly fermentable nature of grain.

Prevention

The best strategy to prevent grain indulgence is to lock all grain behind closed doors and/or in a foolproof, horse-proof container. At all times, do not leave grain containers in areas that a horse may access. However, if this does occur, it is important to obtain immediate veterinary help. Even four or five pounds of grain can be a problem in some individuals. Consumption of fifteen to twenty-five pounds of grain is a definite concern. Sometimes it is difficult to tell exactly how much the horse has eaten, so assume the worst.

Treatment Strategy

If treated aggressively within the first eight to twelve hours, most problems associated with grain overload can be averted.

Your vet will pass a stomach tube and administer mineral oil to limit absorption of endotoxins, which are released from the bowel as gut flora dies due to fermentation of large amounts of grain (starch). Your vet will also medicate your horse with intravenous anti-inflammatory drugs. Frog support may be applied to protect the hooves from laminitis.

Administer a non-steroidal anti-inflammatory medication under the direct advisement of a veterinarian if you cannot obtain professional help immediately.

Recent research indicates that icing the hooves prior to development of overt signs of laminitic pain may prevent the disease from occurring. Cold therapy with ice decreases hoof circulation to deter enzymatic breakdown of the laminar connective tissue in the hooves. Clinical symptoms will be averted or at least lessened with icing, but it should be applied non-stop for the initial twenty-four hours.

Soak your horse's feet in buckets of ice water while waiting to obtain veterinary help. Try to immerse the limbs all the way to the tops of the cannon bones and knees. Standing your horse in a cold stream is useful when ice isn't available.

It is possible that dominant horses ate their fill and moved aside to allow less dominant horses to overindulge as well. There is no point in taking a risk. Treat all horses that could have had access to the grain, even if you think one horse is low in the pecking order and did not necessarily get an opportunity to eat too much.

9.

Fever

If your horse seems lethargic, use a thermometer to check his rectal temperature. An adult horse with a rectal temperature higher than 101ºF likely has a fever, especially when corroborated with other abnormal clinical signs. (See Assessing Vital Signs, page 10.)

It is important to differentiate overheating from increased body temperature related to exercise. An exercising horse may normally have a higher rectal temperature, up to 103ºF, but it should steadily return to normal. But, if a horse is overheated from exercise and strenuous weather conditions, he'll also tend to breathe rapidly and his heart rate will be elevated. In addition, there may be associated abnormal clinical signs if he is suffering from heat exhaustion. (See Heat Stress, page 36.)

How High a Fever?

- In most cases, a fever between 101ºF and 103.5ºF is not in itself harmful unless it is prolonged, but a febrile horse often stops taking care of himself by going off feed and water, potentially developing dehydration or an impaction colic.

- If your horse's fever should rise above 103.5ºF, you'll need to actively help him cool down.

- A fever over 106ºF can be life-threatening, and has the potential to elicit convulsions or seizures, although these consequences are uncommon.

Reducing the Heat Load

Some simple techniques assist your horse in controlling a fever:

- Find an area for your horse that is out of the direct sun—the shade of a tree, behind a horse trailer, or in a barn.

- Make sure there is fresh air moving around the shady area.

- Remove his tack and equipment, or blanket.

- If the weather is windy and cold or wet, it might be better to leave him with at least a light sheet or haunch rug to prevent him from chilling too quickly, especially if he is clipped.

Cooling Down the Fever

You can quickly cool your horse's fever by using the same principle of sweating—evaporative cooling (see Fig. 3).

- Soak your horse's neck and chest areas with room-temperature water by repeatedly immersing a sponge or towel in the water and dousing him with it. Continue this procedure until the skin feels cool.

- Soak primarily the large muscle areas and neck in front of the horse's shoulders. Water applied over his entire body may cool the large haunch muscles of the hind end too quickly, eliciting spasms. (See Tying Up or Myositis, page 39.)

- Every ten to fifteen minutes, recheck the horse's rectal temperature to see how you are progressing in pulling the heat out of his body; you don't want to chill him down too quickly.

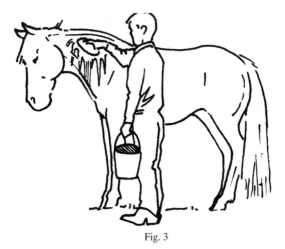

Fig. 3

- If the fever isn't responding, contact a vet immediately and discuss the merits of administering non-steroidal anti-inflammatory medications to contain the fever until you can get professional help.

10.

Coughing

A cough is nature's way of clearing debris or mucus from the airways. It may also be due to a more insidious cause, such as irritation and discharge related to a viral or bacterial infection.

How Significant Is the Cough?

First, try to determine what is causing your horse's sudden cough:

- Gather all vital signs (see Assessing Vital Signs, page 10).

- Check for any discharge from the nostrils and eyes, and evaluate its character.

  - If the discharge is opaque and white, it is likely mucus.

  - A watery discharge is often normal, especially following exercise.

  - If the discharge is discolored (yellowish) or has a malodor, it is likely pus related to bacterial infection.

  - If the discharge is green-tinged, it may simply be food contamination from the back of the horse's throat that mixes with the discharge as he coughs.

- Is the cough stimulated by eating, or by exercise, or does it also occur while the horse is at rest?

- Is the horse able to eat and swallow what he is offered? If not, then he may be sick or may be experiencing choke (see Choke, page 22).

- Does the horse have a normal appetite and disposition? If not, then he may be sick, especially if he has a fever.

- Does the horse appear to be in respiratory distress?

What to Do?

If you establish that your horse isn't in imminent distress or peril as related to choke or a systemic infection, then take some steps to see if the cough will abate easily:

- Shake out all the hay as it is fed, and soak it thoroughly with water to decrease dust and irritants.

- Keep a reasonable distance from other companion horses while riding to eliminate irritation from ground dust kicked up by the hooves.

If it seems the horse may have a contagious disease:

- Isolate the coughing horse from other horses, as far from them as possible.

- Obtain veterinary assistance. This is not necessarily an emergency but should be addressed as soon as possible.

11.

Nosebleed

One odd but not uncommon problem is for a horse to develop a nosebleed, also referred to as epistaxis. Usually, such an incident is of minor significance and resolves itself.

Reasons for a Nosebleed

- Horse hits his head on a firm object or is kicked in the head. Trauma is by far the most common reason to see some blood coming from the nostril(s).

- Sinus irritation from dryness or infection.

- Bleeding in lungs after a hard gallop; referred to as exercise-induced pulmonary hemorrhage (EIPH).

- Guttural pouch infection affecting large vessels in the pouch. This has potentially fatal consequences.

- Ethmoid hematoma, a blood-filled tumor within the sinus that can have eventual fatal consequences but may be managed with surgical attention.

Steps to Take

- Monitor the horse carefully until the bleeding stops.

- Collect all vital signs (see Assessing Vital Signs, page 10) to check for extensive blood loss and to determine if and how quickly you might need veterinary help.

31

- Keep the horse's head elevated if possible. Don't let him graze or eat.

- If the horse allows it, you can pack his bleeding nostril with cotton or a piece of T-shirt to stanch the flow.

The bleeding should slow within about ten to fifteen minutes if the cause is mild and inconsequential, and should stop altogether within thirty minutes.

12.

Dehydration or Shock

Clinical Signs

Mild dehydration of as little as 2 to 3 percent is associated with a decrease in performance, and if exercise continues, more serious dehydration and cardiovascular compromise can lead to shock.

First, check all vital signs to determine if a horse is in trouble or approaching shock (see Assessing Vital Signs, page 10). The horse is likely experiencing significant dehydration and possibly shock if several of the following clinical signs are present:

- Heart rate remains elevated above 80 bpm.

- Respiratory rate may or may not be rapid.

- Mucous membranes are tacky.

- Mucous membrane color is pale or muddy, or brick red.

- Capillary refill time is delayed beyond three seconds.

- Skin, when pinched, remains tented for a prolonged time. (Moistness of the gums and a skin pinch test are only crude assessments of hydration status, and are not always consistent with continuing dehydration.)

- Horse is depressed and off feed.

- Ears and muzzle may be cool to the touch.

- Urine production is scant, absent, or the urine appears very concentrated (darker yellow).

Possible Causes of Dehydration

A horse may become dehydrated for many reasons, but dehydration is most commonly associated with:

- Long trailer ride with minimal access to water.

- Water tank iced over in winter, so horse fails to drink.

- Rigorous or protracted exercise.

- Electrolyte imbalances, especially depletion of sodium through sweat.

- Heat stress (see Heat Stress, page 36).

- Colic (see Colic, page 19).

- Trauma resulting in loss of large volumes of blood.

- Systemic illness, including diarrhea.

Prevention: What to Do if a Horse Won't Drink

The old adage, "You can lead a horse to water, but you can't make him drink," is one frustrating thing about managing a horse. Some horses naturally take care of themselves, and some can be trained to drink, while others simply refuse regardless of what you do.

Here are some possible tricks might entice a horse to drink:

- Offer water in several different types of buckets—galvanized, rubber, and plastic.

- Before taking your horse on a trip, train him to drink water laced with cider vinegar, which you can later use to disguise the odd taste of unfamiliar water.

- Offer a separate bucket of water that also contains electrolytes.

- Offer a wet, sloppy gruel of pelleted feed soaked in water.

- Add 1 to 2 tablespoons of table salt to the gruel, or administer by syringe.

- Soak the hay with copious amounts of water.

- Allow the horse to graze green grass, which has a high water content; but don't graze too long if he isn't used to eating green pasture.

It is good horse practice to continually monitor your horse's vital signs, especially when traveling or exercising rigorously or for extended periods. If your horse's vital signs begin to deteriorate, and especially if your horse has not been drinking well or at all, you should take him to a veterinarian for fluid replacement by stomach tube and/or via intravenous therapy. Besides the tricks mentioned above to entice a horse to drink for prevention of dehydration, it is nearly impossible to force a horse to drink if he is not so inclined. No amount of syringing water into your horse's mouth will make up for the many gallons needed to manage dehydration, and there is always the possibility that syringing water into his mouth by force may cause your horse to aspirate some fluid into his lungs.

13.

Heat Stress

In hot and humid weather, when riding in difficult terrain or for extended periods, or when hauling your horse in the heat of the day, your horse is at risk of dehydration and heat stress (see Dehydration or Shock, page 33). It is important to continually monitor your horse's vital signs (see Assessing Vital Signs, page 10).

Check Vital Signs

- Moistness of mucous membranes.

- Color of gums.

- Capillary refill time.

- Skin pinch test.

- Rectal temperature.

- Heart rate.

- Heart rate recovery: Heart rate should drop to less than 64 bpm within ten to twenty minutes after stopping exercise, and continue to decline to normal range within an hour (see Assessing Vital Signs, page 10).

- Respiratory rate: An overheated or dehydrated horse may have an inversion (respiratory rate higher than heart rate), which should gradually return toward normal with cooling (see Assessing Vital Signs, page 10).

What to Do: Cooling Techniques

A horse with heat stress needs to be cooled down with careful strategies:

- If riding hard, bring the horse immediately to a walk.

- Then stop, dismount and pull off all tack and equipment other than a halter.

- Walk the horse for a couple more minutes to maintain blood flow through the muscles. Abrupt stopping of exercise pools blood in the muscles away from the systemic circulation.

- Light massage of major muscle groups assists the muscle circulation. Caution: Do not massage if the horse is tying up (see Tying Up or Myositis, page 39).

- Offer the horse a bucket of water.

- Move him to a shaded area, preferably one with a light breeze.

- Walk the horse briefly at intermittent intervals to keep the muscle circulation active, dissipating heat from the muscle depths.

- Liberally sponge your horse's head, neck, and legs with cool water, especially over areas with large blood vessels. Apply and scrape away water continuously until the horse's skin feels cool to touch and rectal temperature has dropped to less than 103ºF.

- Apply ice boots to the lower legs.

- If the horse is severely overheated in hot weather, lead him into a pond or creek, or pour buckets of water over him or hose him with full body soaks.

- A horse in a serious heat-stress crisis may need immediate veterinary intervention with intravenous fluids to avoid shock.

An overheated horse should not be cooled too rapidly or he may chill and cramp. Decrease body temperature by about 1ºF over thirty to forty minutes. In hot and humid climates, it may be necessary to apply cold or ice water over the entire body to help cool the horse. In more arid climates, cooling of the large haunch muscles might result in muscle cramping.

14.

Tying Up or Myositis

Tying-up syndrome, or myositis, describes a muscle cramp, usually one that occurs in the haunch or thigh muscles but can occur in any large muscle group. Such cramps are often related to dehydration, electrolyte depletion, and/or heat stress. Sometimes, cramping is also related to hormonal changes (such as estrus in a mare) or a metabolic disturbance or muscle disorder, like equine polysaccharide storage myopathy (PSSM).

Clinical Signs of Myositis

- Shortening of stride.

- Change in disposition and/or willingness to work.

- Sudden onset of rear limb lameness, ranging from subtle to severe.

- Horse refuses to move forward.

- Firm-feeling and/or painful muscle over the haunches and/or along the thigh.

- Colic-like signs: sweating, overt pain, rolling, rapid heart rate, poor heart-rate recovery.

A subtle case of tying up can progress to a serious crisis if a horse continues to exercise. No matter the reason or the severity, a horse with suspected myositis should be stopped from further athletic exertion.

Prevention and Recognition

- Ride only to the level of your horse's capabilities and fitness.

- Administer oral electrolyte supplementation to a horse that works for protracted periods or in hot and humid conditions.

- Allow the horse to drink at every opportunity.

- Monitor frequency and character of urination—dark or discolored urine casts a suspicion of myositis.

- Monitor the gait for soundness—stiffness or lameness often coincides with a bout of myositis.

- A horse with myositis may act like he has colic, and may display similar signs (see Colic, page 19). Evaluate a horse's vital signs to help differentiate myositis from colic (see Assessing Vital Signs, page 10).

First Steps

- Dismount and move your horse to the side of the trail.

- Allow the horse to graze and rest, and to drink if water is available.

- Pull off the saddle and gear.

- Cover the cramping muscle(s) with a saddle blanket or light jacket if there is a chill or a breeze.

- Refrain from deep massage to avoid adding to muscle damage.

- Help cool the horse by sponging his neck and chest, particularly if his skin feels hot and sweaty. Keep water off the cramping muscles of the rear quarters, restricting the soaks only to areas in front of the withers.

• Non-steroidal anti-inflammatory medications such as phenylbutazone or flunixin meglumine should be administered with caution and only under veterinary advisement, as these can cause kidney damage or gastric ulcers in a dehydrated horse. These drugs only help your horse to a limited degree much like a Band-Aid applied to a gaping wound. Many times a horse with myositis needs copious intravenous fluids to combat dehydration and to flush myoglobin (a large protein released with muscle damage) and toxins from the kidneys. Administration of pain-killing medications may enable you to get the horse to help, but do not perceive these to be a cure.

• If the horse is able to walk, slowly proceed along the trail, allowing frequent rest stops. Or, send a friend to get help and a trailer while you wait.

Identify the nearest road access by which a horse trailer and veterinary assistance are able to reach your horse. Discuss this location and the precise course to reach this destination with your companion so people will know where to find you if, after some rest, your horse is able to proceed. Do not deviate from the decided plan. If you are feeling lost in the wilderness or have a poor sense of direction, then simply stay put and wait; let your friend bring help to you. It is best to trailer a horse with myositis to the nearest treatment facility. Have your veterinary location and phone number in hand ahead of time, when possible.

15.

Thumps

"Thumps" describes contraction of the muscles in the region of the horse's flanks. Technically, thumps is referred to as synchronous diaphragmatic flutter (SDF) because each time the heart beats, a muscle twitch is visible or is felt when resting your hand in the flank area. This situation develops most often in a horse that experiences electrolyte and fluid imbalances due to dehydration and loss of electrolytes (salt) through sweating. Salts that are most likely to be depleted in the bloodstream include calcium, potassium, and magnesium ions. This electrolyte imbalance causes the phrenic nerve to become hyperirritable. The phrenic nerve runs across the atrium of the heart to supply nerve function to the diaphragm muscles. As this nerve becomes more reactive, it fires in synchrony with each heartbeat, causing the diaphragm muscles to contract and "flutter."

How to Identify Thumps

- You may see no more than a flutter of the flank muscles as the diaphragm contracts.

- You may only recognize the problem when you put your hand (or a stethoscope) in the area of the flank and feel a twitch.

- A horse may thump only on one side and not the other.

- Thumping may be intermittent, and may come and go.

• More notable cases are visible from a distance, with the flank actively twitching in a rhythmic fashion.

First Steps: What to Do?

• Dismount and remove tack and equipment.

• Assess your horse's vital signs (see Assessing Vital Signs, page 10).

• Stop all exercise.

• Move the horse into the shade if it is a hot day (see Heat Stress, page 36).

• Offer water.

• Offer hay, including a small amount (a flake) of alfalfa, or a mash of alfalfa-based pellets.

• Cool the horse by sponging with water, concentrating on areas in front of the withers, if he is overheated (see Heat Stress, page 36).

• Administer electrolytes by syringe provided the horse has an appetite and otherwise seems okay.

• Call for veterinary help if the horse is depressed, anxious, off feed, or acting colicky (see Colic, page 19).

In most cases if a horse with thumps is stopped from further exercise, the problem spontaneously resolves. In other cases, if a horse has passed a threshold towards more serious ramifications of dehydration and electrolyte imbalances, veterinary treatment is necessary. However, not all dehydrated or exhausted horses show thumps, so it is important to continually assess your horse's vital signs periodically during exercise (see Assessing Vital Signs, page 10).

What Is the Significance of Thumps?

Thumps is a warning sign that underlines the presence of marked fluid and electrolyte imbalances. Hot and humid climates tend to exacerbate the development of dehydration and electrolyte imbalances, but this situation can occur in any horse in any climate. Not only do electrolyte and fluid depletions affect irritability of the central nervous system that controls many muscle functions such as facial and eye muscles as well as the diaphragm, but they also adversely alter normal intestinal motility. Continued exercise complicates the horse's ability to compensate in the face of these losses, and more life-threatening features of exhausted-horse syndrome may surface, including tying-up syndrome, colic, laminitis, heat exhaustion, and/or collapse (see Colic, page 19; Tying Up or Myositis, page 39; Heat Stress, page 36; Acute Lameness, page 76). The time to stop the horse's exercise is long before more serious problems develop and while the horse is still interested in eating and drinking to replenish its energy and fluid losses.

16.

Eye Injuries

Horses are prone to eye injuries, particularly a scratch on the cornea. Injury is usually incurred from running into a branch or obstacle, from rubbing on a tree or bush, or from material blown into the eye on a windy day. Debris also can become trapped in the eye, causing persistent aggravation. With any eye problem, your horse may experience immediate discomfort with visible signs of irritation.

Signs of Eye Injury

- Squinting.

- Sensitivity to light.

- Weeping; watery or opaque discharge.

- Swelling around and/or in the eye.

- Redness and conjunctivitis.

  The tissues around the margins of the eye and beneath the lids are known as conjunctiva. When these become inflamed, as with conjunctivitis, they will appear red and swollen, which is especially noticeable if you open your horse's eyelids even slightly.

First Steps

- Irrigate the eye copiously with water or, if available, use saline solution (purchase a commercial product found on the supermarket shelf, or prepare your own by dissolving a half tablespoon of salt in a quart of water).

- If the horse allows inspection of the eye, look for a foreign body (such as a stick or cactus spine) that may be visible to your naked eye, or at the very least look for an interruption in the smooth surface of the cornea that might indicate a corneal erosion or ulcer.

- Apply ophthalmic ointment (non-steroid type, see below).

- Use a fly mask (if available) to cut down the bothersome ultraviolet glare.

Apply a broad-spectrum ophthalmic ointment every two to three hours to keep the eye lubricated. Do not use any kind of eye ointment that contains a corticosteroid (any ingredient with the suffix "-sone" in the name) as this worsens corneal ulceration. An alternative over-the-counter medication is any human ophthalmic lubricating ointment. Note that wound medications for general-purpose use should never be used in the eye, as they create additional eye damage. Check with your veterinarian in advance regarding safe medications to use in a horse's eye.

MEDICATING THE EYE

1. Rest the outside of your hand that holds the medication tube lightly against the horse's face so your hand moves with the horse's head as he moves.

2. Gently open the horse's eyelids by using the thumb and index finger of your opposite hand.

3. Gently squeeze the tube to place a thin line of ointment or a few drops of solution along the lower lid, preferably without touching the horse's eye.

The degree of discomfort your horse experiences, and the potential for serious eye damage, warrants calling for veterinary attention as soon as possible for any eye injury. Even the most mild eye injury can turn into a serious problem, particularly if infected with bacteria or fungi.

Your initial objective is to make your horse as comfortable as possible and to protect against further damage. Your treatment enables you to see if the problem will resolve fairly rapidly or if professional attention is needed.

More Serious Damage

Sometimes a horse will tear a portion of his eyelid, or may even stab an object into the eye deep enough to penetrate into the inner regions. It is important to cover the eye with a protective bandage until you can obtain professional help.

- Use a saline-moistened, soft pad (such as a sanitary pad, gauze sponges, or a piece of T-shirt) to cover the eye.

- Hold the compress in place with self-sticking adhesive tape. Or, slip a stretchable material, like panty hose, over the horse's face and secure it by cutting ear holes in it.

17.

Allergic Reactions and Hives

A horse can develop an allergy just as people do, with a slow or sudden onset of clinical signs.

Clinical Signs

During an allergic episode, any of the following signs may appear together or alone:

- Hives: This is a typical and preliminary response to more progressive forms of allergy. Also called *urticaria,* hives are localized, raised bumps visible on the skin, variable in size and location. Usually they are firm to touch, but may indent with an impression of your pressed fingertip due to edema within the inflamed tissues (see Fig. 4).

- Depression and possibly a mild fever.

- Swelling in the throatlatch area.

- Swelling in the limbs and/or along the abdomen and sheath or udder.

- Difficulty breathing (see Assessing Vital Signs, page 10).

- Anaphylaxis: Extreme restlessness and sweating, with potential for death.

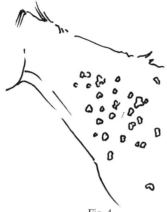

Fig. 4

Common Allergens

A horse may develop an allergy to just about anything, usually following re-exposure to the allergen after a period of time following the initial exposure. Common sources of allergens include:

- Inhaled pollens or molds.

- Biting or stinging insects (see Insect Bites and Stings, page 51).

- Medications, such as antibiotics (especially penicillin) and non-steroidal anti-inflammatory drugs (phenyl-butazone, flunixin meglumine, or ketoprofen).

- Insect repellents.

- Certain pasture plants.

- Feed supplements and especially high protein sources.

- Physical irritants, such as pine shavings, soap used to wash saddle blankets, and antiseptic scrubs.

Managing an Allergic Reaction

What should you do if you find your horse has developed an acute allergy?

- Remove all food and supplements, especially any new element, from the diet other than grass hay.

- Eliminate all medications.

- Cease using fly spray if that is a likely allergen.

- Don't ride or allow the horse to sweat, as this worsens his discomfort.

- Wash blankets and grooming equipment, and be sure to rinse out all the soap.

- Monitor for resolution. If the condition is not resolving steadily within twelve to twenty-four hours, contact a veterinarian for appropriate medical therapy.

In severe cases of an allergic reaction where the airways swell shut and anaphylaxis occurs, it is necessary to treat the horse immediately with epinephrine and corticosteroids as a life-saving measure. This requires rapid veterinary intervention.

18.

Insect Bites and Stings

The most opportune times of year to ride find you in the midst of greenery and blooms, and in the height of insect season. Horses are at similar peril to bites as you are, and some of these biting and stinging insects can elicit significant discomfort for your horse.

Tick Bite

COMMON LOCATIONS TO LOOK FOR TICKS

Usually a tick will bite a horse and latch on until it drinks its fill of blood, and then it drops off. As you groom your horse, you may find an attached tick in various stages of swelling with blood. Ticks seem to prefer the softer areas of skin, although they can be found anywhere on the horse.

Common sites of tick attachment include:

- Around the anus.

- Along the belly and groin.

- Under the chin and throatlatch.

- Behind the elbow.

- In and around the ears.

Ticks can range in size from the size of a sesame seed or smaller to the size of your fingernail when engorged with blood. There may be a single tick, or several, or in the case of "seed" ticks, they may be too numerous to count.

In tick-infested areas, it is useful to apply tick powder to your horse's coat. Most tick powders are formulated for dogs, but check with your veterinarian if a specific product can be used safely on horses, as well. For prevention, brush the powder into the fur, particularly in those areas most attractive to ticks, as described above.

Tick Removal

If you find a tick, remove it as soon as possible, as it has the potential to infect a horse with disease, such as Lyme disease. The longer the tick remains on the horse, the more opportunity there is for disease transmission to occur. Wear gloves or use plastic or a paper towel when handling a tick, and be careful not to get its blood or body fluids on your own skin.

- Grasp the tick behind its head with your fingers or blunt-tipped forceps, and gently pull it out. Do not pull quickly or twist it so that you end up leaving its head embedded in the horse's skin. Examine it after removal to see that its head and mouthparts are intact.

- Once the tick has been removed, manage the wound with general wound care procedures (see Wound Care, page 61).

- Dispose of the tick by burning it, flushing it down the toilet, or placing it in a jar of alcohol.

- If there is concern about a tick-borne disease, then save the tick in a live condition for a month in case testing is necessary. Place the tick on a moistened paper towel and put it into a sealed and labeled vial or bag. Label the container with the date and horse that was bitten, and the geographic area where the tick was found.

Although it may be difficult to release the tick in this manner, it is thought that trying other methods such as smearing it in petroleum jelly or alcohol may cause the tick to "regurgitate" its saliva into the wound, and may increase the likelihood of disease or infection. Applying a hot match to get it to back out is probably not such a good idea, considering that there is a horse attached to one end of the tick and he is unlikely to be happy about a flame near his skin. So, it is best to take your time and proceed with careful, manual removal to pluck it out.

Stinging Insects: Wasps and Bees

When you ride through woods or deep grasses, or alongside old buildings, you may run into a nest of stinging bees, wasps, hornets, or yellow jackets. Not all stinging insects are aggressive, and many will mind their own business if left alone. Bees are the least aggressive of these stinging insects. Be constantly vigilant for the presence of stinging insects, especially when riding past hollow objects near the ground, abandoned buildings, and rocky areas. Bees tend to be irritated by vibrations, so select your path well away from a known hive.

Horses don't like to be stung any more than you do, and are subject to adverse reactions from multiple bites.

STRATEGIES TO AVOID ATTACK

- Wear light-colored clothing, and a light colored helmet since bees seem more likely to attack dark-colored clothing or hair.

- Don't apply sweet-smelling lotions or perfumes or use perfumed shampoo, as these may stimulate bees' keen sense of smell.

- Keep dogs under control so they don't inadvertently run into a hive that then begins to attack.

- Avoid drinking sugary drinks, especially sodas (and even beer), which attract stinging insects, particularly wasps and yellow jackets, to the area.

- If you encounter a group of bees or other stinging insects, refrain from provoking them by swatting at them. The best advice is to flee the area as quickly as possible.

TREATING STINGS

If a horse has encountered a swarm of stinging insects, keep him quiet, and stop further exercise. There are several suggested topical remedies that may or may not help, but may be worth a try as they aren't likely to hurt:

- Cold pack the bite or sting.

- Apply a mixture of baking soda and water to the bite or sting.

- Apply calamine lotion to the area.

- Apply tobacco to the bite or sting.

In cases of multiple bites or stings, the horse may need veterinary intervention, which will include systemic anti-inflammatory treatment and antihistamines.

Spider Bite

Despite the enormous variety of spiders lurking in dark corners, two common ones are of most concern to your horse: the black widow and the brown recluse. These spiders are often found in woodpiles, barns, and sheds.

A brown recluse is also referred to as the "fiddleback" or "violin" spider. When a brown recluse bites, it sets off a localized reaction in the surrounding skin. The black widow can elicit both a localized and systemic reaction. Only the female black widow bites.

CLINICAL SIGNS OF SPIDER BITE

- Inflamed and necrotic area of tissue in a local area.
- Very sensitive to touch over the bite.
- Itching in the bite area.
- Hives

TREATING SPIDER BITES

A spider bite on a horse may elicit considerable localized discomfort and hives, but is not usually a critical emergency crisis. Have a veterinarian examine your horse in a timely fashion to relieve discomfort with anti-inflammatory medications and antihistamines, and to remove affected tissue so the extent of necrotic tissue doesn't spread. In the meantime, manage the bite as with regular wound care (see Wounds Care, page 61), and try some of the anti-sting suggestions above.

19.

Wild Animal Encounters

When riding or camping in the wilderness, one of the exciting experiences is being among wild animal residents. It is uncommon to encounter large wild animals, but it is possible to catch them unawares. Some of these are, of course, large predators that can stimulate a horse's flight reflex. A horse may be frightened into fleeing the campsite, or if you are mounted and on a trail, you could be thrown while your horse runs off (see Lost Horse, page 94).

Avoiding Large Predators

Precautionary measures may save you a lot of grief and headache later. Some things you can do to avoid unwanted encounters with large predators:

- Know the time of year and seasons when certain predators might be likely to pass through the woods.

- Check with the local forest service, park rangers, and wildlife officials as to the frequency of sightings of bear, mountain lions, or wolves in the areas in which you plan to ride.

- In camp, hoist human food, garbage, and horse grain high into the trees to keep bears from accessing these tasty treats and to keep from attracting them in the first place. Or, enclose all potential bear food in bear-proof metal containers.

- Set up human sleeping and horse picketing areas a distance away from the eating area.

- When riding in bear country, place bells on your horse's saddle and breast collar, and purposefully make a lot of noise (talking and singing) as you progress through the woods.

- Be vigilant of your surroundings.

- Carry pepper spray with you at all times.

- If you are adept and comfortable with a gun, carry a high-caliber weapon and know how to use it in the event of a predator attack. (Know if your horse will tolerate you firing of a weapon from his back before you do so.)

An Encounter

If you encounter a large predator on the trail, stop your horse and keep him standing quietly. Stay mounted. Don't be tempted to turn your horse and flee, as this could spark a predator's instincts to chase. Don't advance toward the predator, as this could be perceived as a confrontational threat and might stimulate an attack. Give the bear or lion ample space to pass without coming into close range of you and your horse.

Dogs often deter large predators from entering your campsite and alert predators to the presence of humans and horses so they have time to leave the areas. However, dogs are also at risk of an attack or of stimulating an attack. Keep your dogs close and under obedient voice control or on a leash.

Small Animals

In general, small animals present little risk to your horses unless there is a high incidence of rabies in the area. To protect your horse, be sure to immunize annually against rabies when riding in an area especially populated with skunks, raccoons, and bats (see Chart of Vaccination Recommendations, page 106).

20.

Snakebite

Whether riding in the desert country or the prairies of the West or in the woods of the East, rattlesnakes are always a concern. Most rattlers are timid and retiring, and a horse's pounding hooves vibrate the ground sufficiently to send a snake on its way unless the horse steps on it. More commonly, a horse browsing in the grasses inadvertently sticks his nose on a sleeping snake and may be struck (see Fig. 5).

The Dangers of Snakebite in Horses

Unlike dogs or people, horses do not succumb rapidly to the effects of rattlesnake venom. In fact, the majority of snakebites are "dry," meaning that no venom is injected. A big problem is the injection of anaerobic bacteria (Clostridium sp.) into the bite wounds, with associated risk of infection. The other concern with a snake strike is the rapid swelling that accompanies the bite. If the bite is on the face around the nostrils, swelling has the potential to obscure the airways and make breathing difficult.

First Steps

Generally, you'll have plenty of time to get your horse to veterinary help. In the meantime:

- If the wound is on the muzzle, slash the puncture holes with a pocketknife to make them bleed and to allow for swelling. Try the best you can to do this over both

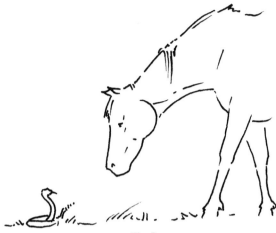

Fig. 5

fang marks, but don't risk getting struck by an angry horse.

• Make your way to the trailer, and veterinary assistance.

• If you have antibiotics with you in your emergency kit, start the horse on an appropriate dose (recommended in advance by your veterinarian) to forestall infection.

• A dose of non-steroidal anti-inflammatory medication, like phenylbutazone or flunixin meglumine, helps to control inflammation, pain, and swelling.

• If the horse is having difficulty breathing and is demonstrating distress, it may be necessary to insert the end of a large plastic syringe case or a four- to six-inch piece of garden hose or similar rigid material into the inner reaches of each nostril to ensure passage of air. The swelling associated with the snakebite generally affects only the external tissues of the muzzle, and not the inner portions of the airways or throat.

21.

Wound Care

Any number of injuries can occur when the thin skin on a horse's legs encounters a solid obstacle, such as a branch, tree, root, rock, or jumping obstacle, or is hit by one of the horse's hooves. Several possibilities exist when a horse is wounded: 1) a superficial abrasion, 2) a puncture, or 3) a full-thickness cut or laceration. If a large vessel is injured, there could be hemorrhage associated with the wound. (Hemorrhage is unrelenting bleeding that isn't clotting or stopping its flow.)

First Steps

- Reach a safe place.

- Dismount and assess the damage.

- If the horse allows it and excess bleeding isn't a problem, clean the wound of debris and as much as possible, as described below.

- Apply an antibacterial ointment.

- Cover the laceration with a clean, nonstick dressing.

- Tape the dressing to the leg with elastic tape.

- Move the horse to a location free of obstacles and as little dirt as possible.

Abrasion

An abrasion is the mildest form of wound and does not extend past the superficial layer of skin; only the hair and a shallow portion of the skin are missing. Such a wound is not likely to become infected, and needs only to be thoroughly cleansed and have ointment applied to keep the tissues from drying out. If a leg abrasion is extensive and the horse lame because of it, then a bandage might provide tissue support and improve comfort for your horse while keeping the tissues soft and pliable.

Non-Bleeding Wound or Laceration

1. Clean the wound with salt water (and antiseptic scrub if available) as best as possible to remove the bulk of contaminants.

2. Cover the wound with antibiotic ointment on a non-stick dressing.

3. Or, cover the wound with sugar and povidone iodine mixture ("sugardine"), which acts as an effective antiseptic.

4. Or, soak gauze compresses in saltwater solution (mix a half tablespoon of salt to one quart water) and lay them over the wound.

5. Or, seal the top of the wound with Superglue®. Apply in small spots like stitches, leaving large areas between dabs of glue. Use only a limited amount, as it is difficult to remove later to properly clean and treat the wound.

6. Systemic antibiotics may be administered under the advisement of a veterinarian.

7. Regardless of the depth or extent of a wound, make sure your horse is current on his tetanus immunization.

Bleeding Wound

1. Secure a bandage snugly around the bleeding wound.

2. Elevate your horse's injured leg if he'll allow it and will stand quietly.

3. Place firm finger or hand pressure directly over the injury.

4. If ice is available, apply ice directly over the wound when covered by a bandage.

5. Check the horse's vital signs (see Assessing Vital Signs, page 10) and monitor for shock (see Dehydration or Shock, page 33).

Dealing with Hemorrhage

Resist the urge to unwrap and look at the injury to see if the bleeding has stopped. Some large arteries require thirty to sixty minutes to clot. A horse can lose up to two gallons of blood before he suffers a life-threatening cardiovascular crisis and shock.

If the bleeding still won't stop with direct bandaging:

• Use a hemostat or the pliers in an all-purpose tool to grasp the spurting vessel, clamp it tightly, and give it a tiny twist. Blood vessels run side by side with nerves, so beware that your horse might react suddenly if you grab or touch the wrong structure.

- If you don't have an all-purpose tool, hemostat, or bandaging supplies on hand, then rip off the bottom portion of your T-shirt and form into a bandage compress. Bind this to the leg with duct tape, or tear the ends of the T-shirt and tie them in a knot around the leg.

- Elevate the leg if possible, apply pressure, and then be patient and wait.

- If the bleeding still persists, then make a temporary tourniquet (using a piece of latigo from your saddle, the bridle's leather throatlatch, or a shoelace) wrapped snugly above the wound. To avoid tendon and circulatory damage, don't leave a tourniquet on for more than fifteen minutes.

Rope Burn

When a horse entangles his leg in a rope, the friction created as he attempts to free himself will create a "burn."

- Immediately cut the rope with your pocketknife so your horse doesn't continue to inflict damage.

- Then, assess the damages.

- Immediately take him to a creek to immerse his leg in cold water, or apply ice. This will soothe the pain for a while and will slow the thermal injury.

- Apply silver sulfadiazine cream, which is particularly useful for burn wounds or any equine laceration. For the short term, if nothing else is available, lip balm might provide some relief by lubricating the injury.

- Lightly bandage the wound to keep dirt from grinding into the painful tissues. An alternative for a bandage is a torn piece of T-shirt with the ends tied into a knot, or on the lower leg, pull a tube sock over the hoof to the knee.

Thermal injury to the tissues causes them to slough more tissue in the days following a rope burn. You'll have plenty of time to get your horse back to the trailer and home for veterinary attention.

Puncture Wound

Any penetrating object can create a puncture wound, as can any blunt trauma. With blunt trauma, the tissues separate, sometimes forming an open tract through the tissues that can become infected just as would a puncture. It is sometimes difficult to tell if a tiny wound or abrasion extends deeply into underlying structures. Unless clearly obvious, assume all wounds are punctures until this can be ruled out.

- Clean the wound thoroughly.

- Apply topical antibiotic ointment.

- Bandage to avoid further contamination.

- Seek veterinary attention to determine the depth and extent of the injury.

Joint or Tendon Sheath Penetration

Penetration of a joint or tendon sheath has crippling and potentially life-threatening consequences. If you suspect any involvement, even a tiny puncture, of a joint or tendon sheath, cover the wound to protect against further contamination and then get your horse to veterinary help as quickly as possible.

Speared by a Tree or Branch

A horse can bully his way through obstructions with his sheer weight and size. Just because a horse skewers his torso or belly on a sapling, tree branch, or board fence doesn't mean he will stop moving forward at that instant. The result of such brute force may be a terrible-looking wound with a long and large piece of the forest impaled in your horse. Where this material is wedged determines the practicality of its removal. Keep in mind that it could have entered some large blood vessels inside the horse, making removal a serious problem. On the other hand, the only way you may be able to move the horse to a safe place is to remove the object. Just be ready for anything when you do. (Use good restraint and stand to the side of the horse when attempting to remove any foreign body. Grasp the object as close to the horse's body as possible and pull firmly without twisting.) These situations arise no matter how hard you wish them away. There is no recipe for handling this event, but just be mentally prepared and use good common sense. Then, apply basic first aid care for wounds.

22.

Bandaging Primer

There are many ways to apply a bandage, and you may find a method that works better for you, although differing a bit from the following recommendations. However, these guidelines give you a starting point for safe bandaging of the lower leg.

Lower Limb Bandage

1. Clean the leg of all debris and dirt.

2. Scrub the wound if possible (see Wound Care, page 61).

3. If the wound has a hanging flap, try to position the flap flush against the leg and bandage it with light pressure to keep it in place.

4. Apply water-soluble antibiotic ointment to the wound, and cover this with a nonstick dressing.

5. Wrap one to two layers of cotton or gamgee around the cannon bone and/or pastern. Apply smoothly without wrinkles, and with uniform pressure.

6. Optional: secure the cotton into place with conforming roll gauze firmly but not tightly applied.

7. Using self-adhesive bandage material, start taping at the middle of the leg, roll the tape up the limb to the top of the cotton, then work your way back down

to the bottom, then up again to end the tape in the middle of the cannon bone when possible.

8. As you wrap the self-adhesive bandage material, pull the tape loose from its roll as you come across the front of the leg, and lay it gently across the back of the leg. This minimizes the possibility of binding the tendons with an overly tight bandage.

9. Apply the bandage so that it encompasses the entire lower leg, from the top of the cannon bone to just above the hoof line (se Figs. 6a and 6b).

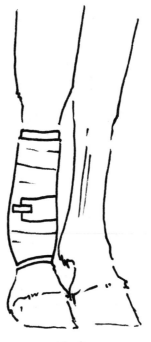

Fig. 6a

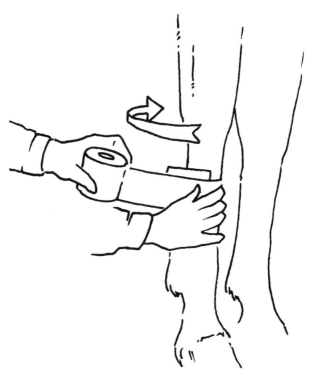

Fig. 6b

10. Leave cotton or gamgee sticking out above and below the margins of the self adhesive bandaging material.

11. Secure the ends of the bandage with white adhesive tape or another type of self-adhesive sticky tape, but do not apply either too tightly or circumferentially around the leg.

Hoof Bandage

If you need to bandage the hoof for any reason, the best method is to use a hoof boot. If a synthetic hoof boot is not available, then you can make a bandage for the foot:

1. Apply a non-stick dressing or povidone-soaked piece of cotton over the area of concern.

2. While holding up the foot, lay a square of cotton or gamgee over the entire bottom of the hoof, allowing the cotton to stick up around the sides of the hoof and behind the heel bulb.

3. Use self-adhesive bandaging material, and begin to tape it over the bottom of the hoof.

4. Continue to bandage by layering it over the bottom of the hoof, around the bottom edge of the hoof, and then in a figure-8 pattern across the back of the heel bulbs. This figure-8 method helps keep the bandage from slipping.

5. Over the front of the hoof, if possible, keep the bandage material below the coronary band, or at least do not apply too tightly across the coronary band.

6. Once this bandage is secure, apply duct tape across the bottom (sole) of the hoof to minimize wear of the bandage material. Reapply duct tape as necessary.

7. Use blunt-end bandage scissors to later remove the bandage.

Splinting for Possible Fracture or Serious Limb Injury

Once you have the lower leg bandaged as above, it may be necessary to splint the leg to immobilize a possible fracture or tendon laceration. As a general rule, the joints above and below a fracture must be stabilized and immobilized.

If the fracture is of the front cannon bone, then bandaging will need to encompass the knee and below the fetlock—that is, everything from just below the elbow to just above the hoof. If the fracture is located in the pastern area, then the entire foot, pastern, and fetlock need to be encased in bandaging and splint.

1. Bandage the area of injury as described above, incorporating the joints above and below the fracture site or injury.

2. Apply more layers of cotton (one to two rolls) over the bandaged leg to provide ample padding, or wrap a pillow around the entire circumference of the leg

3. Secure this padding with conforming roll gauze and/or self-adhesive tape, pulling very firmly as you wrap so there is no chance of loosening. Remember, the objective is to hold the bones securely in a fixed position, and with sufficient padding you are not likely to compromise blood circulation. Fracture stability also decreases the horse's pain.

4. Lay a rigid, rodlike splint (a 2x4 board, a straight branch, a broomstick or rake handle, or a piece of PCV pipe cut longitudinally in half to form a bivalve piece) along both sides (inside and outside) of the leg, with the ends extending to at least the bottom surface of the hoof or sticking slightly down below the bottom of the hoof. Make sure the tops of the splints extend past the joint above the fracture line.

5. Secure the splint sticks with self-adhesive bandaging.

Put in an emergency call to your veterinarian. Arrange for immediate transport to a veterinary hospital for radiographs and surgery.

23.

Hematoma or Seroma

A hematoma is a blood-filled swelling that develops following an impact trauma, such as a kick or a fall. Bleeding in underlying muscle or soft tissue collects in a swelling just beneath the skin and subcutaneous tissue layers. The dimension of the swelling ranges from golf ball to grapefruit sized. Sometimes, the pocket of fluid pools with yellow serum rather than blood, in which case it is called a seroma. As you push lightly on such a swelling, it may feel like a water balloon, with the fluid bouncing in waves beneath your finger.

First Steps

In most cases, there is little urgency in acquiring veterinary treatment to manage hematomas and seromas in the initial day or two. Steps you can take:

- Application of ice packs slows the bleeding and limits swelling in the immediate period after the trauma.

- It is best to wait a couple of days for the bleeding to stop before draining the swelling, especially if the hematoma or seroma is a result of a torn muscle belly.

- Confine the horse for the first few days to limit additional muscle and fascial trauma that might stimulate more bleeding.

It is best to have these swellings drained eventually, as blood or serum provides a nutrient medium for bacteria to proliferate, which could create infection. Also, it takes a long time for the fluid to reabsorb if not drained, and this usually leaves an unsightly lump and large blemish. Your veterinarian will determine the best timing to open and drain the fluid. A hematoma or seroma usually heals uneventfully following drainage and treatment.

24.

Girth Galls and Saddle Sores

A saddle sore on your horse can easily put you out of the saddle for weeks to months and modify your plans for a riding trip. A girth or cinch that fits poorly can bunch up along the girth area and create a friction rub.

Prevention

- Use girths and cinches that have a smooth surface.

- When necessary, pad a cinch or girth with fleece so it slides more easily across the skin.

- After you buckle the girth or cinch, stretch your horse's front legs forward to release trapped folds of skin.

- Make sure the girth or cinch is neither too snug nor too loose. A loose girth allows a saddle to shift from side to side. A tight girth pinches and compresses thin skin, creating bruises and chafed areas.

- Use saddle pads that wick moisture away from the skin and won't trap too much heat beneath the saddle.

- Make sure your saddle fits well without pressure points or shifting.

Treatment

As with any wound, immediate care starts it on its way to healing (see Wound Care, page 61).

- Clean the wound with antiseptic scrub to expose fresh, bleeding tissue.

- If the wound is fresh, a cold pack or ice helps limit the inflammation; after the initial couple of days, warm packs may give added relief.

- Apply drying products like Desitin® or Preparation H® if the wound is weeping serum, or use water-soluble ointments to keep the sore pliable.

- Use fly spray around the wound, so insects don't irritate the traumatized area.

- Avoid using caustic powders, as these increase scar tissue and thickening.

If you need to ride your horse out of the wilderness, you can take the following precautions to limit skin damage:

- Use gunny sack material over the girth or cinch to protect a girth gall.

- Cut a hole in a thick fleece pad if the sore is beneath the saddle.

This removes direct pressure from the wound, but do not be lulled into thinking it will effect a cure. Girth sores won't go away until the pressure and chafing are removed entirely. The key to treating girth or saddle sores is to give the tissue sufficient time to rest and heal

25.

Acute Lameness

Is There Really a Lameness Problem?

If you think your horse may not be moving quite right, gather some information:

- Check for a stone or rock that might be wedged in the clefts of the frog, and also check for thorns or cactus spines lodged in tender, soft tissue.

- Have a friend jog the horse out in a straight line and see if you notice any missteps.

- Jog the horse in circles or put him on a longe line and see if the lameness worsens.

How Lame Is Lame?

The American Association of Equine Practitioners (AAEP) has developed a grading system to classify the degree of lameness a horse is experiencing:

- Grade 0: Lameness is not perceptible under any circumstances.

- Grade 1: Lameness is difficult to observe and is not consistently apparent, regardless of circumstances, such as moving the horse under saddle, on circles, on inclines, or on a hard surface.

- Grade 2: Lameness is difficult to observe at a walk or when trotting in a straight line but consistently apparent under certain circumstances, such as carrying weight (of a rider), circling, inclines, or hard surface.

- Grade 3: Lameness is consistently observable at a trot under all circumstances.

- Grade 4: Lameness is obvious at a walk.

- Grade 5: Lameness produces minimal weight bearing in motion and/or at rest or a complete inability to move (see Fig. 7).

There are various levels within each grade, but this gives you something to work with when communicating with a vet or in making the determination of how serious the problem might be. If your horse is Grade 4 (lame at a walk) or Grade 5 lame (not willing to put the limb on the ground), you'll need immediate veterinary attention.

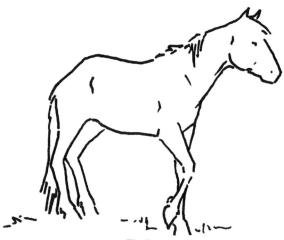

Fig. 7

MODERATE WEIGHT-BEARING LAMENESS (GRADES 1, 2, 3)

The first three lameness categories describe a horse that is able to walk without overt lameness and is willing to trot when asked, albeit lame to different degrees. In all circumstances, it is best to stop riding activities and to confine the horse, which reduces the likelihood that activity will worsen the injury.

SIGNIFICANT WEIGHT-BEARING LAMENESS (GRADE 4)

This lameness is visible as the horse walks or turns, and may be due to any number of problems, such as a foot abscess, a joint injury or degenerative arthritis, a torn ligament, or tendon injury. The horse may only touch his toe to the ground for support as he is asked to move, but if he'll put any weight on the limb at all, the lameness is classified as Grade 4, not Grade 5.

NON-WEIGHT BEARING LAMENESS (GRADE 5)

When a horse is referred to as being "three-legged lame," this is what is meant by the Grade 5 designation. In such cases, the horse will not under any circumstance put any weight on his leg, and if asked to move, he will hop on the opposite limb with the injured leg held off the ground, without allowing it to touch the ground.

Some possible problems of serious import that will render a horse so lame he can barely walk or refuses to touch the foot to the ground include:

- Fracture.

- Foot abscess or nail puncture.

- Joint or tendon sheath penetration and/or infection.

- Soft tissue injury, such as with a ligament or tendon tear.

- Cellulitis (an acute infection within the muscles or connective tissue of a limb, usually subsequent to trauma).

Is There Swelling?

Sometimes you are able to localize the lameness problem if there is discernible swelling of the limb. Look carefully and compare each leg to its opposite to see if one is abnormally larger than the other. Not all lameness problems are accompanied by swelling, particularly if the injury is located somewhere within the hoof.

Sometimes the leg is diffusely swollen, especially if there has been an interval between injury and when you notice that there is a problem. In these cases the swelling may have already gravitated to the lower portions of the limb, causing the swelling to encompass considerable portions of the leg. Under these circumstances, it is more difficult to determine the source of the injury.

If there is discrete swelling:

- Ice pack or cold hose the area for ten to fifteen minutes at a time, two or three times per day.

- Apply a compression bandage (if you are comfortable doing so) to the lower limb if swelling is located below the front knee (carpus) or hock (see Bandaging Primer, page 67).

- Reapply this bandage daily or following every cold therapy application.

- Confine the horse until you can obtain veterinary counsel as to the significance of the injury.

- Administer a non-steroidal anti-inflammatory medication under the advisement of your veterinarian.

Nail Puncture

If you find a nail in your horse's foot:

- Mark the spot with indelible ink or take a photo of it before you pull out the nail. This enables your veterinarian to pare away directly over the penetrating hole for evaluation and to establish drainage.

- Clean the hoof thoroughly to remove all dirt, debris, and manure.

- Check to see if there is a soft or tender spot on the back of a heel bulb or along the coronary band where an abscess may be trying to drain. This may develop if the nail has been in place for a day or two and infection is well under way.

- Clean the hoof thoroughly with water and a scrub brush to remove all contaminants and dirt.

- Soak the foot in a clean bucket of warm water with as much Epsom salts as you can dissolve in water, and add enough tamed iodine solution to approximate the color of weak tea.

- Or, soak the foot in a running creek if that is all that is available.

- After soaking for ten to fifteen minutes, bandage the foot or place it in a synthetic boot to keep it clean.

- Soak the foot two or three times daily.

- Apply cotton or a towel over the entire foot to prevent material from contacting the injury.

- Wrap the hoof in a bandage or place in a synthetic protective boot.

- Get veterinary attention as soon as possible for your vet to open the puncture and administer appropriate medical care relative to the location and depth of the nail puncture.

Stone Bruise or Foot Abscess

You cannot always know what is exactly wrong without veterinary diagnostics, but you may see some obvious indications that your horse has a bruise or abscess. A bruise may appear as a pink discoloration on the sole of the foot, and an abscess may create a tender spot along the coronary band or heel bulb or may be actively draining from such a soft tissue location. Or, an abscess may be identified as a soft spot on the bottom of the sole that once opened, will drain tarry-looking pus. If it is obvious or suspected that your horse's problem is a stone bruise or a foot abscess, then proceed as above with a nail puncture, and use a synthetic boot to protect the horse's foot from further trauma.

Pulled Tendon or Sprain

On occasion a horse will slip or may jam a leg in an abnormal position while still moving forward, and he may acutely pull a tendon or sprain a joint.

- Compare one leg to the opposite leg and look for any sign of swelling or asymmetry.

- Feel down the tendons and squeeze gently to determine if there is any discomfort. Compare one leg to the other as some horses are overly responsive to even mild touch and this doesn't necessarily mean that your touch or pressure elicits true pain.

- Stand your horse in a cold, running creek or in a bucket of ice water for thirty minutes or so to minimize the inflammatory response. Periodic icing over the initial forty-eight hours continues to help.

- Administer non-steroidal anti-inflammatory medication (phenylbutazone or flunixin meglumine) only under advisement by your veterinarian to help arrest the inflammation.

Confinement and sufficient rest time are important to minimize reinjury and to allow healing.

26.

Loose or Lost Horseshoes

Horseshoe problems are common anywhere you ride. A shoe may be loose, lost, or may be sprung or twisted yet still remain attached to the hoof. This impedes forward progress since your horse can't put his foot down flat on the ground.

Sprung or Twisted Shoe

Although you may not have shoeing tools on hand, there are methods that help you remove a shoe.

- Use the file on a medium- or large-sized multipurpose tool (such as a Leatherman®) to file away the clinches on the outside of the hoof.

- Then pry the shoe off a little at a time with pliers, banging the shoe back down with a rock to expose the top of each horseshoe nail.

- Pluck each loosened nail out using the pliers. Check that a nail isn't broken off in the hoof wall, and if so, try to pull it out. A broken nail left in the hoof doesn't usually cause much of a problem.

- Or, if you have a shoe-pulling pliers specific for the job of removing shoes, then first file off the clinches as above. Then, using the shoe-pulling pincers, grab the rear of one rear branch of the shoe and rotate the pliers towards the opposite side of the toe. Repeat for the other side, again pulling diagonally toward the opposite toe. This means your pull is toward the center of the foot, not toward the outside of the foot. Do these steps gently without violent twisting or yanking.

Loose Shoe

As you ride, you may hear the jingle of a loose shoe that is in danger of detaching from your horse's hoof. It is best to stop and attempt a fix before the shoe falls off or gets sprung, or your horse steps on one of its nails (see Figs. 8a, 8b, and 8c).

- Place your horse's foot with a rock directly beneath the head of one of the loosened nails, then take the screwdriver part of the multipurpose tool and pound it with a round rock directly over the nail clinch. It should seat down nicely after a few bangs.

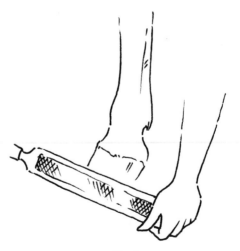

Fig. 8a

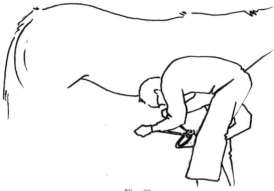

Fig. 8b

- If you don't have a tool, then bang directly on the clinches with a rock while holding another rock firmly against the head of the nail.

- A synthetic boot that fits over a loose shoe can be applied to the hoof to avoid losing the shoe altogether.

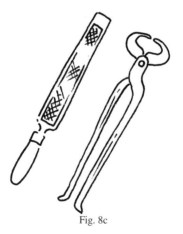

Fig. 8c

Missing Shoe

In instances where a shoe is lost or you have had to remove it, the hoof is then susceptible to bruising and trauma. Usually, a horse isn't too uncomfortable with a lost hind shoe, but he will be less sore if you can protect a bare front foot.

- You should ride with a synthetic boot (such as an Easyboot® or Old Mac® boot) affixed to your saddle. The boot should be sized to fit your horse's unshod front foot.

- If you haven't got a hoof boot, you could wrap the foot with Vetrap and duct tape secured over some soft material like a piece of t-shirt. Then, lead your horse down the trail slowly and return to the trailer. Try to find soft footing when possible, and reapply duct tape as necessary.

Stepped on a Nail

Sometimes when a horse loses a shoe, he doesn't just walk out of it, but rather it twists and pulls several nails free before the entire shoe falls away from the foot. In such a case, there is a chance the horse will step on one or more of the sharp nails or clips (if present) to puncture the bottom of his foot (see Acute Lameness: Nail Puncture, page 80).

27.

The Cast or Entrapped Horse

When a horse is placed in any enclosure, there is a possibility that he will roll up against the wall and be unable to get up because he can't get his trapped hind legs beneath him to push up. A horse thus stuck is referred to as being cast (see Fig. 9).

In other instances, an older horse with degenerative arthritis in the hind end may have difficulty pushing himself off the ground if lying on the side with the bad leg. In effect, this horse is cast or stuck even though there may be no physical obstacle in the way of him getting up.

And, in yet other situations, a horse's legs may be caught in a fence or become entangled in wire, unable to safely move.

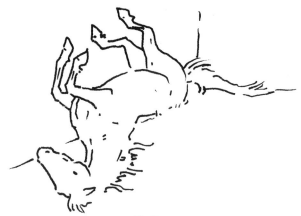

Fig. 9

First Steps to Free a Cast Horse

The first thing to do is to remain calm. If you've got a friend on hand, that is best, but you can rescue a cast horse on your own by following some precautions:

- Place a halter and lead rope on the horse so you have some measure of control once he starts to get to his feet.

- Gather up several soft ropes.

- Encourage the horse to lie quietly while you affix a rope loop to each of the lower front and hind legs, placing a loop over each pastern closest to the ground.

- Or, each person grabs onto the pastern of the lower front and hind legs closest to the ground. Only do this if the horse is tractable and you can stay out of harm's way.

- At all times, stay behind the horse, out of range of the moving arc of any of his legs or head.

- Do not put yourself in a trapped position in a tight enclosure. Make sure you always have a way out in case the horse struggles as he tries to get to his feet.

- With your friend, together pull on the ropes or his lower legs to roll the horse onto his other side, or to roll him out of his position where he is stuck against the wall or fence.

- If conscious, he will likely roll his head and neck on his own when you roll him over, so you needn't worry about guarding his head.

- Then, he should be able to get up on his own.

FURTHER MEASURES

If the horse is struggling while you try to extricate him from his trapped position, have someone positioned in a kneeling position behind his neck, with a knee placed firmly on the horse's neck while pulling his nose back toward the person's lap. This prevents a horse from trying to rise, giving you time to place a loop on his pasterns and begin to roll him over.

If the horse continues to struggle, you may be able to settle him some by placing a blindfold to fully cover both eyes. Often, the horse will quiet down with a blindfold, allowing you to reassure and soothe while working to extricate him.

If the horse still can't get up after you have rolled him over, then you will need more manpower or horsepower to help. If the horse is attempting to rise on his own, but can't quite make it, sometimes you can give him that little extra boost by lifting up on his tail, particularly if two or three people help him get his hindquarters lifted. Grab his tail close to where it attaches to the body, and pull straight up without bending the coccygeal vertebrae at the base of his tail, and in no circumstance should you pull so hard that you strain your back.

If this doesn't work, then try edging a blanket or strong band (such as a tow strap) beneath his girth and side, and then help him up by lifting the band with a tractor bucket.

If you have no tractor nor manpower to help, or if the horse still won't get up but seems otherwise okay, contact your local fire department and see if they are willing to come and help. Veterinary assistance may also be necessary to sedate a thrashing horse to enable people to help him.

Entangled in Wire or a Fence

If your horse is trapped in a fence or becomes entangled in wire that wraps around his leg, this is a job for wire cutters or your multipurpose tool. The first priority is to keep the horse calm by speaking softly and keeping your cool. Then, after ensuring that you are not in range of having any part of yourself in contact with the horse should he blow up while you are attempting to free him, start cutting the wire away from the horse's trapped leg. Pay attention at all times to what the horse is doing and how he is reacting, and be prepared for a sudden eruption.

You may need veterinary assistance and sedation to safely move the horse so he is no longer trapped or cast.

Once the Horse Is on His Feet or Freed

Once the horse is no longer trapped or cast, check his vital signs and look for any wounds that need attention (see Assessing Vital Signs, page 10; Wound Care, page 61).

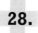

28.

Smart Constraint

There are some basic tenets to follow to ensure that your horse doesn't part company from you while out riding. Some situations are unpredictable, so if you do get thrown because your horse spooks or bolts, you may be forced to let go of the reins to protect your body parts. Then, you've got a horse on the loose.

Precautions on the Trail

Ride with at least one other person in case you are thrown, not only for your safety but also to enable quick recovery of your horse. Being a herd animal, your horse will tend to stay with the other horse(s) and is less likely to run off. And, if he does, a friend can follow him on horseback to catch up with him.

On a camping trip, it is sometimes tempting to ride the saddle horses while leaving the packhorses to follow without constraint. If there is more than one packhorse loose on the trail, a couple of them may venture off on their own, content with each other's company, but now separated from the group. Or, one of the horses might try to pass a saddle horse and create a commotion, or pose a hazard to you or your riding horse. For horses that won't stay in line, it is best to lead them on a lead line to avoid pile-ups on the trail.

Part of the wilderness experience means pausing on the trail to enjoy the view, eat lunch, take photographs, or go fishing. Tie your horse securely (by rope and halter) to a strong tree, making sure he can't get tangled in the branches with his lead line, or catch his leg over a rope. Use a leather or breakaway-style halter in case your horse does break loose; rope halters or nylon halters will not give under pressure when snagged on a solid object, and that result could be disastrous.

Methods of Containment

In camp, there are several excellent methods of securing your horse.

HIGHLINE

An overhead tie line (highline) is a stout rope secured between two strong trees, or between two horse trailers or a combination of tree and trailer.

Find a location with relatively level and solid footing, free of natural hazards. Separate each horse by a safe distance that prevents kicking or entanglement—at least twelve to fifteen feet. Tie each lead line so the horse cannot get his head much lower than his chest. When you are able to monitor the horses, you can lengthen the lines to release their heads to graze or lie down. The horse's nose should just barely reach the ground so he won't entangle his leg in the rope.

PICKET LINE

A picket line is a length of rope usually thirty feet long, connected to a stake hammered deeply into the ground or tied to the base of a big tree. Drive the stake straight down into the ground, as it is more easily pulled out if set at an angle. Attach the rope from the stake to a single hobble on the horse's leg.

The horse can then walk in a large diameter to graze, and can lie down at will. Make sure he doesn't wrap the line around the base of a tree, thereby shortening the line so much that he gets stuck. Don't be tempted to picket to a down tree or log, as a strong horse can run with these in tow, and that is not only frightening to the horse, other horses, and people, but is also potentially disastrous.

HOBBLES

Hobbles are invaluable in managing horses on camping trips so they can take advantage of available pasture to feed. Be sure to train your horse to hobbles or a picket line at home before encountering the real situation. That gives both you and your horse a measure of confidence in these kinds of restraints.

Stagger the horses left loose in hobbles at any time, so all are not loose together. Keep one or more of the dominant mounts tethered to a stout hitch or highline in camp while the others feed. Affix a cowbell to a ribbon around each horse's neck to keep yourself (and the other horses) constantly informed of their location and presence.

CORRAL

Portable corral panels safely enclose your horse when you are camped near your truck and trailer. Make sure that you double-check all gates and clips, as a bored horse is able to let himself out if you forget to secure the latches.

Don't ever rely on using an electric fence enclosure, because a horse can easily run through it. A "hot" fence deters a horse from getting near it, but when he does, it is hardly a barrier for a 1,000-pound animal with a startle and flight reflex.

29.

Lost Horse

On wilderness camping episodes, at least one horse may get loose and go missing. Knowing some basics about horse behavior helps:

- Many times the horse will go just a short distance, within sight.

- Grab a container of grain and start toward your horse, but don't approach directly. Try to go around to the side so you can then approach from his front rather than coming up from behind. He'll be less likely to feel "herded" away, and you may be able to turn him back toward camp if he just won't be caught.

- Some horses are leery of a halter, so use common sense in hiding it within your clothing. Walk carefully, and stop if it looks like your movements may stimulate him to move away. This process may seem like a dance, at times. Croon softly to him so he knows where you are, letting your voice lull him to allow your approach.

- When you reach to put the halter on, move carefully, first slowly putting your arms or the lead line over his neck so he'll feel "caught."

The Missing Horse

If your horse has taken off for the backcounty , you'll have a bit more of a project to find him. Although you may not be able to see him, he may be close at hand, able to see you through the thickets and trees, so search in near areas first. If it is evident that the lost horse has gone missing far from camp, take a few moments to get organized.

When you begin looking for your horse, remember a few caveats:

- A frightened horse tends to go uphill, especially when hampered by hobbles.
- He'll tend to go back the way he came, but not necessarily following the trail.

Supplies to Bring on a Search

As you prepare for your search, plan on being gone for a while. Bring all necessary supplies:

- Flashlight with fresh batteries.
- Rain gear.
- Drinking water.
- Lead ropes.
- Halter.
- Grain or enticement in a bucket or feedbag.
- Energy bars for yourself.
- Wire cutters or an all-purpose tool.
- First aid supplies for a laceration.
- Map of the area, preferably one with topographical markings so you'll know how to traverse tough terrain without running into a cliff.

- Cell phone in case you have cell service. Bring a fully charged battery and fully charged spare.

- Your vehicle keys to give to someone, so they can retrieve your truck and return to pick up the horses when found.

Some of this seems like common sense, but you'd be surprised how much you forget in the heat of a panic. Many horses are found by tracking their hoof prints. Stay off the path they have followed so you don't muddy the picture in case you need to retrace those steps. Ideally, while hunting for your missing mounts, you'll be in the saddle, riding the horse that was left securely tied in camp. If all are missing, then wear good walking shoes!

Still Missing

If you still cannot find your horse after hours of searching, you might consider hiring a small plane or helicopter to scan the general area of the backcountry where your horse got lost. It is important to implement this as early in the search as possible, particularly if your horse is garbed in saddle, bridle, or halter, to find him before he becomes dangerously snagged. Set up communications with ample ground support to expedite recovery of horses seen from the air.

30.

Basic Restraint

When you need to administer emergency first aid, the horse must cooperate to allow treatment. Handling the horse relies on effective control and decisive actions by the handler.

- Control the horse with a halter that fits well and a soft lead rope with a reliable snap on the end. Use gloves when necessary to prevent rope burn. A makeshift halter can be constructed by using a length of rope, first looped around the neck and secured with a bowline knot; then pass another loop through the neck loop to be placed over the nose.

- When possible, have a capable handler hold the horse while you examine or minister to the horse.

- The handler should always stand facing forward, to the side of the horse's head, with a firm grip on the lead line, holding the lead line no more than about three feet from the snap.

- When working on a front limb, the handler should stand on the opposite side of the horse from the examiner.

- When working on the rear area, the handler should remain on the same side as the person working on the horse, and if the horse threatens or menaces the person in any way, the handler should immediately turn the horse's head toward both handler and examiner, thus swinging the horse's hindquarters away from the examiner and out of range of a kick.

- No one should stand directly in front of the horse at any time.

- If a horse is down on the ground, in all cases people should stay well out of range of the arc of swing of any leg or the horse's neck, preferably working from behind the horse's back.

If more restraint is necessary, some devices are useful to distract a horse:

- Apply a twitch to the upper nose. Hold the shank of the twitch perpendicular to the ground and the horse's nose so as not to twist his nose into abnormal positions. In a pinch, a twitch can be made with materials

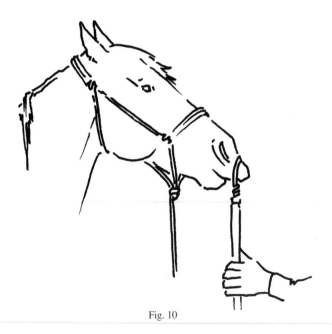

Fig. 10

on hand. Apply a loop of baling twine over the upper nose and twist it to clamp down and distract the horse (see Fig. 10).

- Place a lip chain over the upper gum line. Make a homemade lip chain by using a piece of rope or baling twine, placed beneath the upper lip and over the upper gum line. Try to use materials that won't break easily if the handler needs to pull on it, or the horse throws his head with force.

- For a skin pinch, the handler takes a large bunching of neck skin in hand and squeezes.

- An ear hold should be done in a reasonably kind manner by gently pulling the ear down, and holding it firmly.

- A blindfold that completely covers both eyes sometimes makes a horse stand perfectly still for a short time.

All restraint devices and techniques must be used with caution as any horse may violently explode when so restrained, without any forewarning. All restraint devices should be used with the utmost kindness and respect for the horse, and not to torment or abuse in any way. If a horse doesn't respond favorably to restraint tactics, it is best to forego attempts at treatment and get the horse to a veterinary professional as soon as possible to avoid injury to horse or handler.

31.

First Aid Kit for Horses

Stocking a Basic First Aid Kit

In a first aid kit, you will have supplies that are readily available over the counter. Other supplies that are helpful may need to come from your veterinarian. You should be proficient in the use of any prescription medications and use them only under advisement from your veterinarian.

STORAGE CONTAINER

- Purchase a plastic container with an airtight lid. This serves as both a storage vessel and a scrub vessel. On the side of the container, identify how full the container will be with one quart of liquid by marking a line with indelible ink.

- Include pre-measured baggies, each with a half tablespoon of salt to add to one quart of water for cleaning wounds or irrigating an eye.

WOUND CLEANING MATERIALS

- Disposable razor or scissors for hair removal.

- Gauze sponges for scrubbing.

- Antiseptic (povidone iodine or chlorhexidine) solution to add to saline for rinsing and irrigating wounds. Use

10 ml povidone iodine or 20 ml chlorhexidine per liter (or quart) of salt water.

- Antiseptic (povidone iodine or chlorhexidine) surgical scrub for scrubbing wounds.

- 35 cc or 60 cc syringe for wound or eye irrigation.

- Disposable gloves.

WOUND TREATMENT MATERIALS

- Topical, water-soluble antibiotic ointment to apply to wounds.

- Diaper rash ointment (Desitin®) for saddle sores or rope burns.

- Superglue®.

- Hemostat.

- Flexible rubber tubing or thin strip of leather to use as tourniquet.

BANDAGING MATERIALS

- Sterile, nonstick dressing.

- Roll gauze.

- Cotton or gamgee.

- Self-adhesive stretchable bandage material.

- Sticky veterinary wrap bandaging material or ace bandage for pressure bandaging.

- Bandage scissors.

OTHER ESSENTIALS

- Rectal thermometer, five-inch large-animal type.

- Stethoscope to count heart rate and to check intestinal sounds.

- Multipurpose tool.

- Hoof pick.

- Tweezers or forceps.

- Duct tape.

- Hoof boot.

- Fly repellent, in squeeze packets to fit in saddle bag.

- Flashlight with fresh batteries.

PRESCRIPTION MEDICATIONS

- Non-steroidal antibiotic eye ointment.

- Broad-spectrum oral antibiotics and oral dose syringe.

- Non-steroidal anti-inflammatory systemic medication (phenylbutazone, flunixin meglumine, or ketoprofen) for pain and swelling.

- Short-acting intramuscular sedative for pain relief. (Your veterinarian must be comfortable with your handling and use of this medication before dispensing it. And, be aware that if your horse is insured and someone other than a veterinarian administers such medication and a problem develops, the insurance company is under no obligation to honor your policy.)

- Epinephrine to counteract allergic reaction.

OPTIONAL ITEMS

- Instant hot and cold packs.
- Towels.
- Plastic baggies.

Items to Carry on Your Saddle

- Sponge.
- Hoof pick.
- Hoof boot fit for front hoof.
- Stethoscope.
- Multipurpose tool.
- Sharp folding knife to cut rope if horse gets entangled.
- Small pocket flashlight with fresh batteries.

32.

Equine Vaccinations

Keeping your equine partner "as healthy as a horse" relies on immunization strategies. Most vaccines immunize against viral infections, but a few bacterial infections also present effective vaccine choices.

Vaccination Strategy

For a horse that has never received vaccines before:

- The horse should receive a two-series vaccine protocol, the second injection given three to five weeks following the first, or per the manufacturer's recommendations.

- A foal will begin its immunizations based on the vaccination schedule of the mare prior to foaling and the relative risk of disease in the area. Discuss particulars with your veterinarian.

- It will take about two weeks following the second injection for the horse to develop immunity to protect against that specific disease.

- A booster will be given one to two times per year, depending on the disease type, geographical and seasonal factors, relative risk of exposure, and the duration of protective coverage incurred by each vaccine.

- Booster horses two to four weeks prior to intended travel or competition.

Necessary Vaccines for All Horses

- Tetanus—given annually.

- Eastern and Western equine encephalomyelitis (EEE and WEE)—given annually, or twice a year if living in year-round mosquito environments.

- Venezuelan encephalomyelitis—only necessary for horses in states or traveling to states adjacent to the Mexican border.

- West Nile virus—given annually, and depending on which vaccine used, may need to give a six-month booster in areas with year-round mosquitoes.

Recommended Vaccines for All Horses

- Equine influenza virus—given twice yearly.

- Equine rhinopneumonitis virus—given twice yearly to all horses, and for pregnant mares at months five, seven, and nine of pregnancy with products labeled for use in pregnant mares.

Optional Vaccines Used in Endemic Areas

- Strangles—given annually in high-risk areas.

- Rabies—given annually in high-risk areas.

Chart of Vaccination Recommendations

Disease	Initial Series	Booster Frequency
Equine Encephalomyelitis (Western & Eastern)	2 injections, 4 weeks apart	Annually or every 6 months if high risk
Equine Encephalomyelitis (Venezuelan)	2 injections, 4 weeks apart	Annually in states bordering Mexico
Tetanus	2 injections, 4 weeks apart	Annually
West Nile Virus	2 to 3 injections, 3 to 5 weeks apart or 1 injection if using chimera vaccine	Annually, or every 6 months if high risk and not using chimera vaccine
Equine Influenza	2 to 3 injections, 4 weeks apart (do not begin sooner than 8 to 9 months of age if mare was immunized prior to foaling)	Every 6 months
Equine Rhinopneumonitis (Herpes virus)	2 to 3 injections, 4 weeks apart	Every 6 months or for pregnant mares, booster at 5, 7, and 9 months of pregnancy
Strangles	2 intranasal vaccines, 3 weeks apart	Annually in high-risk situations
Potomac Horse Fever	2 injections, 3 to 4 weeks apart	Efficacy questionable at this time
Rabies	1 injection	Annually in high-risk areas
Equine Viral Arteritis	Use 3 weeks prior to breeding	Annually in high-risk situations or mare is to be bred to EVA-positive stallion
Botulism	3 injections every 30 days during last trimester of pregnancy	Last trimester of pregnancy: Every 30 days in high-risk areas
Rotavirus	3 injections every 30 days during last trimester of pregnancy	Last trimester of pregnancy: Every 30 days in high-risk areas

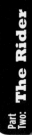
{Gilbert Preston, MD}

1.

First Response

In the backcountry you can't call 911. Yourself and your companions are all you have to rely on. This can be frightening, especially if you have never been responsible for the immediate care of a seriously injured or ill person. If you attend first aid courses, CPR classes, and avalanche awareness seminars, you will feel more confident and be more effective in a wilderness emergency situation. You must immediately decide if the victim is alert or unconscious, if she is breathing, and if her circulatory and nervous systems are functioning normally. Once you have made these critical decisions and acted appropriately, take a few deep breaths. Then move on to your evaluation of less critical conditions.

Evaluating the Victim

1. Ask the victim, "Are you okay?" If she cannot answer, check to see if she is choking or has stopped breathing. Is she clutching her throat and making high-pitched or grunting sounds? If so, treat for choking (see Choking, pages 109–111).

2. If the victim responds with a coherent answer, then the victim is conscious, breathing, and has a pulse. You must ask permission from a conscious victim before administering first aid. The victim has the

right to refuse care. Disregard this wish only if she appears delirious and self-destructive.

3. If the victim is not choking but is unable to answer, check to see if she is breathing and has a pulse; see the ABCs (pages 110–112). If the victim passes the ABC checklist, CPR is not required. If the victim fails the ABC test, administer CPR (pages 112–114).

4. If the victim is breathing and has a pulse, but is not conscious, check for head injury (pages 125–128) and spinal injury (pages 128–131).

5. Is the victim bleeding, either inside her clothes or from an obvious wound? Expose the wound, if necessary, and apply direct pressure and treat for bleeding (pages 132–135).

6. If she is experiencing shortness of breath, paleness, and squeezing chest pain, treat as if she is having a heart attack (pages 121–122) and be prepared to administer CPR (pages 112–114).

7. If the victim is not bleeding and is not experiencing heart attack symptoms, and she has passed the head injury and spinal injury checklists, evaluate for signs of injuries that do not pose an immediate threat to life. Treat injuries or conditions as described in the appropriate chapters.

8. When your evaluation and treatment are finished, decide if the victim requires evacuation from the wilderness and, if she does, can she walk or ride out safely or should someone go for help? If the decision is made to self-evacuate, then continue to monitor the victim for a change in her condition that could require more immediate evacuation. See Getting Help (pages 115–116) to decide if evacuation is necessary.

2.

CPR
(Cardiopulmonary Resuscitation)

Cardiopulmonary resuscitation (CPR) is used to revive a person who is not breathing and/or has no pulse. Cardiopulmonary arrest may occur in the backcountry as a result of massive trauma (a fall from horse, an avalanche); an extreme lowering of the body's temperature (hypothermia); near drowning; heart attack; an extreme allergic reaction to plant, reptile, or insect toxins (anaphylaxis); or excessive loss of blood (shock). The most common reason a child may need CPR is that breathing has stopped due to choking, asthma, near drowning, or severe allergic reaction. (See page 111, if you suspect the airway is blocked.)

Successful revival of a person whose heart and lungs have stopped working requires compression of the chest to force blood from the heart in order to restore circulation, and rescue breathing to supply oxygen to the system. A person who has suffered massive head or chest injuries, or who has had extreme blood loss, cannot be resuscitated in a wilderness setting by CPR alone. A person whose heartbeat is not restored after thirty minutes of CPR is extremely unlikely to survive (exceptions would be someone who has suffered cardiac and respiratory arrest due to severe hypothermia or cold-water near drowning).

The rules for doing CPR in the wilderness are different than they are back in town. In the backcountry, the safety of rescuers and other group members takes precedence over what might be considered standard medical management in an urban setting. Before giving first aid treatment, make sure you can do so without risk of further injury to the victim, yourself, or your companions. If the victim is in a dangerous location, do not begin treatment until both victim and rescuers are moved to a safe place.

CPR requires professional instruction and regular practice. Consult your local chapter of the American Red Cross or a nearby search and rescue unit. You cannot learn CPR by reading a first aid book. The discussion and diagrams below are intended to refresh your memory if you have not practiced CPR in some time.

If you have reason to believe a person has suffered cardiopulmonary arrest due to trauma, you must stabilize the victim's head and neck before you lift his chin or move his head for your airway check and rescue breathing (see Fig. 11).

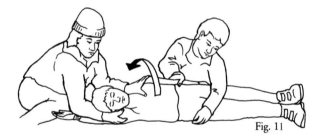

Fig. 11

ABCs (Airway, Breathing, Circulation) for Adults and Children

AIRWAY

1. As soon as the victim is in a safe place, check for breathing: watch for chest movement, listen for breath sounds, feel for breath from the nose or mouth. Allow ample time—ten seconds is typically enough—for careful observation.

2. If there are no signs of breathing, or if breathing is weak or shallow, establish an airway with the head tilt–chin lift maneuver and give two rescue breaths, one second per breath:

    • Keep chin tilted up, but neck straight.

    • Be careful not to force the victim's head back if there is any chance he has suffered a neck injury (see Spinal Injury, pages 129-131).

    • Pinch nostrils with thumb and first finger.

    • Cover victim's mouth with your mouth and blow air slowly into his mouth. Pause for several seconds between breaths to allow air to flow out of his chest.

    • If victim's chest does not rise and fall with rescue breaths, reposition the head and try again. If rescue breaths still do not go in, open the mouth and remove any visible obstructions. If victim does not breathe spontaneously after you have cleared the upper airway, repeat rescue breaths. If chest still does not rise and fall, the lower airway may be obstructed, and you will need to begin chest compressions (see CPR below) even if the heart is beating. After thirty chest compressions, attempt rescue breathing again. Repeat chest compressions and attempt rescue breaths as necessary until the airway is cleared.

BREATHING

If the victim does not breathe spontaneously after airway is cleared, resume rescue breathing.

CIRCULATION

Check for a pulse at the carotid artery and look for other signs of circulation that include breathing, coughing, or any movement. If there is no indication of circulation after ten seconds, begin chest compressions (start CPR).

Note: If a child or adult is hypothermic and has no signs of circulation or breathing, do not attempt chest compressions as it may cause immediate cardiac arrest. Hypothermic victims should receive rescue breathing only.

Adult and Child CPR

1. Roll victim onto his back on a firm surface. Move the body as a single unit, keeping neck and spine straight if he has suffered trauma.

2. Bare the victim's chest and place heel of hand on breastbone in center of chest (about two to three inches below the V where breastbone and collarbones meet; see Fig. 12). Use a CPR shield if it is available.

3. Place your other hand on top of first hand and interlock fingers. Keep shoulders, arms, and hands in a straight line with your weight over them (see Fig. 13).

4. For adult or child, a clearly visible depression of the breastbone must occur. Compress the chest thirty times at a rate of one hundred compressions per minute.

5. After each set of thirty chest compressions, stop long enough to provide two mouth-to-mouth breaths of one second each.

6. Continue chest compressions and mouth-to-mouth, as above (see Fig. 14).

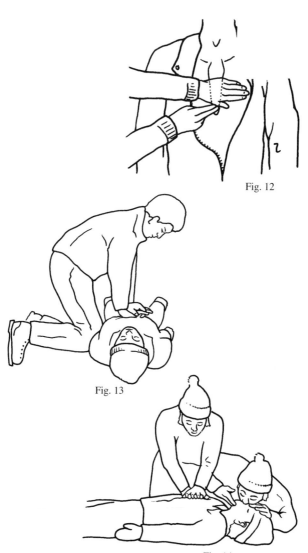

Fig. 12

Fig. 13

Fig. 14

7. Check for carotid pulse and other signs of circulation every few minutes; take about ten seconds to be sure.

8. If no signs of circulation after thirty minutes, consider stopping CPR if the victim has not been turned over to definitive medical care. (For hypothermic victim, continue to give rescue breathing without chest compressions as noted earlier.)

3.

Getting Help

A wise backcountry rider knows that few destinations are worth the price of life or limb. Poor judgment on your part may put the lives of rescue professionals or volunteers at risk. You have a moral obligation to evacuate yourself and companions before you have gone past the medical point of no return.

When to Stabilize the Victim On Site and Get Help

Get help right away if someone is experiencing any of the following:

- Dizzy spells or fainting spells.

- Pulse rate that remains above 110 beats per minute at rest for more than an hour.

- Difficulty catching breath even when at rest.

- Progressive weakness at rest, or with only mild exertion.

- Declining awareness of her surroundings.

- Loss of consciousness for more than two minutes, especially after a head injury.

- Pain so severe she simply cannot continue.

- Chest pain that is very clearly not due to an injury to the muscles or bones.

When to Self-Evacuate, if Possible

Self-evacuate if any of the following conditions are present:

- Vomiting or diarrhea that gets worse despite basic first aid treatment.

- Inability to hold down liquids.

- Vomiting blood or bleeding from the rectum.

- An infection that is spreading.

- A psychological state that endangers the person or other members of the group.

Always err on the side of safety. When in doubt, GET OUT or GET HELP!

Getting Out Safely

Rescues in the wilderness are rarely a matter of brave rangers rappelling from a helicopter. They are most often dirty, sweaty, extremely uncomfortable, and dangerous affairs for everyone, especially the victim. If the injury is severe, and self-evacuation is not an option, send two of your party for help, and have one or two members of the party remain to monitor the injured person for life-threatening changes. If the injury is minor and moving the victim won't make the problem worse, then it is safe to self-evacuate. Whenever possible, those who go for help should not travel alone.

Once out, contact trained emergency rescue personnel: an injured rider may not be able to ride out to safety and it takes six physically fit adults to move an injured person on a litter one hundred yards over easy ground (more than six on difficult terrain). The safety of the rescuers and the injured person's companions takes precedence over what might be considered otherwise ideal medical management.

4.

Shock

Shock occurs whenever the flow of blood, with its payload of oxygen and nutrients, falls below the amount required to maintain bodily functions. In the wilderness, shock is seen most commonly as a result of major internal or external blood loss, burns, severe dehydration, severe allergic reactions, insulin reactions in diabetics, or heart attacks. Shock is life threatening, requiring the highest level of rapid evacuation, up to and including helicopter rescue.

Signs of Shock (All Causes)

- A catastrophic drop in blood pressure.

- Rapid, shallow breathing.

- A sudden rise in pulse rate, which feels weak, shallow, and "thready."

- Pale, cool, and clammy skin.

- A decline in alertness.

Treating Shock

1. Stop all bleeding as quickly as possible (see Bleeding, pages 132–134).

2. Lay victim down, flat on the ground, with legs elevated no more than ten to twelve inches (as long as

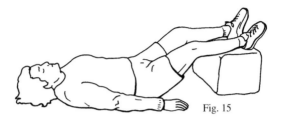

Fig. 15

there is no sign of head injury, serious leg fracture, or spinal injury; see Fig. 15).

3. Keep victim warm with ground pad, blankets, sleeping bags, or extra clothing.

4. If the victim is alert and thirsty, with no evidence of head injury or abdominal injury (and can swallow without vomiting), she may drink clear fluids, including oral replacement salts in water or sport drink. Fluid intake is adequate when plentiful, clear, colorless urine is produced.

Evacuate all shock victims as soon as possible, using safe procedures. See Getting Help, pages. 115–116. For severe allergic reactions (anaphylactic shock), see pages 167–168.

Insulin Shock (Hypoglycemia)

The dosage of insulin a diabetic routinely uses at home may dangerously lower the blood sugar due to the increased exercise level required for backcountry travel, and can lead to insulin shock. Insulin shock in the backcountry looks much the same as other forms of shock, and the initial treatment is the same (see page 117). A person suffering from insulin shock requires a promptly administered dose of a rapidly absorbed carbohydrate (glucose) to bring bodily functions back in balance. If you suspect someone is in insulin shock and follow the steps outlined below, you will cause no harm whether or not they are diabetic, and you may very well save a life.

SIGNS OF INSULIN SHOCK

- Suspect insulin shock in an unconscious stranger if signs of shock are present, and there is no obvious major trauma or blood loss.

- Victims of insulin shock often develop the symptoms slowly and may appear cool, clammy, and drunk, unable to make sense.

TREATING INSULIN SHOCK

- If you suspect insulin shock, treat the victim for it. If the victim is able to swallow, provide a sweet drink, juice, or candy. If the victim is unable to swallow, sugar or honey smeared inside the mouth will be quickly absorbed. This treatment will not harm a victim in shock for other than diabetic-related reasons. Try two or three tablespoons to start; depending on how low the victim's blood sugar is, you may need to provide three or four tablespoons, or more.

- People with diabetes must recognize their personal insulin shock reactions, and carry their glucose monitoring kit and supplies for appropriate treatment with them. If you are a diabetic, teach your companions how to use your blood sugar monitoring kit, and share your insulin reaction information and supplies of quick-acting glucose with trip companions. Check with your doctor before heading into the backcountry for advice regarding adjusting your insulin dosage, diet, and other factors.

- If you are the companion of a diabetic, carry backup commercial glucose gel or sugar packets. Smear small quantities of the gel or granules of sugar inside the mouth or under the tongue of a victim in insulin shock; one or two packets of commercial carbohydrate-rich gel will provide 100 to 200 calories, as would packets of sugar.

5.

Chest Pain

Many medical conditions can cause chest pain that mimics the pain of a heart attack. The typical heart attack victim is a middle-aged smoker, but people under thirty can and do have heart attacks. Chest muscle pain, anxiety symptoms, and indigestion or heartburn are the most common causes of chest pain in otherwise healthy adventurers in the wilderness.

Heart Attack

A heart attack requires immediate medical attention. Many conditions that are not life threatening can imitate a heart attack, but there is often no way to sort them out in the wilderness. If a person shows any of the signs listed below, alone or in combination, she or he must be considered to be having a heart attack until proven otherwise by professional medical evaluation.

PREVENTING HEART ATTACKS

A healthy diet, regular exercise, and consulting a physician before strenuous exercise can reduce the risk of a heart attack in the saddle. If you are over forty, smoke, or are obese, and have not physically conditioned yourself for riding in the wilderness, a pre-season checkup makes good sense.

SIGNS OF HEART ATTACK

- Pain or pressure in the center of the chest that begins with physical exertion, often described as a crushing or squeezing, unbearable pain.

- Pain that radiates from the chest or upper abdomen up to the neck, jaw, or throat, or down one or both arms.

- Any chest pain accompanied by shortness of breath, sweating (usually on the face and head), nausea, or vomiting.

- Any chest pain accompanied by an overwhelming sense of impending doom.

- Any chest pain that is accompanied by fainting or lightheadedness.

TREATING HEART ATTACK

1. Remain calm and keep the victim as emotionally and physically calm as possible.

2. Be prepared to check the ABCs and provide CPR (pages 110–114).

3. One-half an adult aspirin may buy time for evacuation by slowing the blood-clotting process. Nitroglycerin tablets used according to a doctor's instructions will buy time for a person with known heart disease.

4. Evacuate as soon as possible to professional medical attention. Do not attempt self-rescue for a person you suspect is having a heart attack. GET HELP!

Soreness (Musculoskeletal Chest Pain)

Musculoskeletal chest pain is pain in the muscles and tissues of the chest rather than in the heart or lungs. It is caused by overuse or strain of the muscles and ligaments.

SIGNS OF MUSCULOSKELETAL CHEST PAIN

- Aching and soreness due to exercise or injury.

- Constant, achy tenderness, aggravated by movement of the affected area or finger pressure on the affected area.

- Lasts two to four days.

TREATING MUSCULOSKELETAL CHEST PAIN

1. Treat as a muscle strain, with ice and heat (see RICE page 139).

2. Aspirin, acetaminophen, or ibuprofen may be used to relieve pain. Follow instructions on label.

Chest Pain Due to Stress

Stress can cause anxiety in anyone at any time. Rides for which you are physically or psychologically unprepared are far more likely to induce stress reactions than those for which you are well prepared. Do not allow your enthusiasm to bully your common sense.

SIGNS OF CHEST PAIN DUE TO STRESS

- A sense of pressure in the chest or a feeling of suffocation.

- Numbness and tingling of the lips or fingers.

- Trembling.

- Rapid heart rate.

- Rapid, shallow breathing.

TREATING CHEST PAIN DUE TO STRESS

1. Stop for rest.

2. Offer or get reassurance and support of companions.

3. Prescription medications that do not suppress respiration and have no abuse potential may be useful additions to the wilderness first aid kit. Consult a physician if you are prone to anxiety symptoms. (See First Aid Kit for Riders, page 173, for alternative medications.)

6.

Head Injury

Head injuries are among the most severe wilderness emergencies because they can cause injury to the brain. Head injuries commonly occur during a fall from a horse or from a blunt-force blow to the face and neck. Serious brain injuries are a primary cause of accidental death, and riders are at a high risk. A great number of these injuries and deaths can be prevented or reduced in severity by wearing a well-fitting riding helmet that meets ASTM/SEI standards.

See Spinal Injury (pages 129–131) before treating a victim with a head injury, since the two types of injury frequently occur at the same time. If the victim with head injury has lost enough blood to be in shock (see Shock, pages 117–120), search for other internal or external injuries. If there are none, the victim's shock is most likely caused by damage to the spinal cord.

Low-Risk Head Injuries

Head injuries in which there is a blow to the head and a loss of consciousness or change in state of alertness for no more than one or two minutes, and after which the victim is alert, speaking normally, and walking around normally, are considered low-risk head injuries.

SIGNS OF LOW-RISK HEAD INJURY

- Confusion or loss of memory about the accident that led to the blow for no more than one hour.

- Scalp and facial lacerations which may bleed profusely, but do not penetrate the skull or facial bones.

- "Goose eggs" that swell impressively but are not associated with deformities or depressions of the skull.

TREATING LOW-RISK HEAD INJURIES

1. Stabilize the neck before the victim is evaluated or moved (see Fig. 11, page 110). Once the neck and spine are stabilized, the victim must be logrolled into position for evaluation. Logroll the victim onto a sleeping pad or other insulation to keep her off the bare ground. Her head and neck must remain in line with one another until she passes the spine check (page 130).

2. Apply pressure with a bulky dressing to the bleeding scalp or face and a cold compress to the "goose egg" (see also Wounds, pages 132–135).

3. There is no need to evacuate people with low-risk head injuries because by definition these people are up and walking around under their own power, and in every way appear to be their usual selves within the hour. Nevertheless, these people still require close observation for twenty-four hours.

High-Risk Head Injuries

Victims who receive a blow to the face, head, or neck and are unconscious for more than two minutes are at high risk for serious brain and/or spinal cord injury. The longer they are unconscious, the greater the risk of more severe brain or spinal cord injury. If any of the signs of severe head injury or skull fracture listed below appear, the victim requires immediate evacuation. High-risk head injury justifies helicopter rescue.

SIGNS OF HIGH-RISK HEAD INJURIES

- Inability to wake the person up.

- Changes in level of alertness (difficulty remembering name, location, day of the week).

- Nausea and vomiting that persists or appears worse an hour after the initial blow.

- Headache that gets worse.

- Personality changes.

- Unusual irritability.

- Changes in vision.

- Changes in balance or coordination.

- Slurred speech.

- Convulsive seizures.

- Greatly enlarged pupil on one side and not the other.

- Black and blue marks ("raccoon eyes") surrounding one or both eyes.

- Black and blue marks ("Battle's sign") behind the ears or on the upper back of the neck.

- Clear or blood-tinged fluid draining from the nose or ears (unless there are cuts, scrapes, or a nasal fracture in the area).

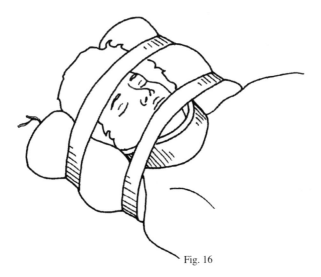

Fig. 16

TREATING HIGH-RISK HEAD INJURIES

1. Immobilize the victim's neck, even if she is alert (see Fig. 16).

2. Once the victim's neck and spine are immobilized, logroll her into position for stabilization, keeping her head and neck in line with one another until you are sure she does not have a spinal injury.

3. Get help ASAP. Do not attempt to self-evacuate the victim (see Getting Help, pages 115–116).

7.

Spinal Injury

The physical forces that can cause a head injury can also cause a fractured neck. People with a low-risk head injury can nevertheless have a serious neck and spinal injury. All trauma victims must be thoroughly evaluated for both head and neck injuries. An unstable fracture in the neck can change position and cause irreversible damage to the spinal cord, which can result in permanent paralysis or death.

Signs of Head and Neck Injury

The neck (cervical spine) must be stabilized (temporarily made unable to move) in all trauma victims before the victim is evaluated. Ideally, one rescuer should stabilize the victim's neck, while a second carries out the evaluation. Once the neck and spine are stabilized, the victim must be "logrolled" into position for evaluation (see Fig. 11, page 110) so that his head and neck remain in line with one another until you are sure he does not have a spinal injury. Logroll the victim onto a sleeping pad or other insulation to keep him off the bare ground. In cold weather, cover the victim with extra clothing and sleeping bags to prevent loss of body heat. If the victim and rescuers must move to a safe place before the evaluation, then the victim's neck must be immobilized (see Treating Spinal Injury, page 131) before he is moved.

A trauma victim's head and neck must be immobilized (see Fig. 16, page 128), and the victim evacuated immediately if:

- He is unconscious, or not fully alert.

- He appears intoxicated.

- He has sustained other injuries that are painful (dislocated joint, fracture of arm or leg, abdominal injury, chest injury), which may mask the pain of a fractured neck.

- There is any complaint of localized, severe pain in the neck or back.

- He reports pain when you carefully run your finger down his spine from the bottom edge of the skull to the bottom of the lower back using direct finger pressure.

- He reports numbness, tingling, or loss of sensation anywhere on the extremities, body, or face.

- He cannot wiggle his toes or move his feet, lower and upper legs, hands, fingers, upper and lower arms, or facial muscles.

Note: On rare occasions, trauma victims who "pass" this checklist still turn out to have an unstable fracture of the spine when they reach definitive medical care. The decision to allow a victim who has "passed" this exam to walk or ride out must be made on an individual basis. If the decision is made to immobilize a suspected neck injury in a safe location, while members of the party go for help and others stay behind with the victim, there can be little criticism of the decision. If the party, and the "passed" victim, decide to walk or ride out of the backcountry and not await professional rescue (assuming no other incapacitating injuries are found), then keep in mind that a fractured vertebra may still be present, and the sudden appearance of any of the checklist items during self-evacuation requires immediate neck immobilization and emergency evacuation.

Treating Spinal Injury-Immobilization

(See Fig. 11, page 110, and Fig. 16, page 128)

1. One rescuer temporarily stabilizes the victim's head and neck between his hands and arms.

2. A second rescuer places a neck collar around the victim's neck. The collar can be improvised by rolling up clothing, cutting the end from a foam sleeping pad, or using a backpack hip belt. The collar should be taped or tied to itself to keep it in place. This immobilizes the neck from forward and backward movement.

3. Place rolled-up items of clothing, such as jeans, sweaters, or jackets, alongside the victim's head and neck to prevent head movement from side to side. These braces or soft splints must be long enough to reach from the level of the collarbone to above the victim's ears.

4. Use duct tape or bandage material to secure the splints by taping them across the forehead and chin so that the head and neck cannot move from side to side. Do not obstruct the airway as you secure your splints.

5. Send for help to evacuate the victim. Maintain immobilization while waiting for, and during, evacuation.

6. Maintain normal fluid intake to prevent hypothermia and shock. Oral fluids, enough to keep the urine clear, are okay if the victim is alert, awake, and not vomiting frequently.

First Aid Tip

Carry a flexible plastic straw in your first aid kit to allow the neck-injured victim to sip drinks without moving or choking.

8.

Wounds

Bleeding Wounds

Minor cuts are those without bone, tendon, or joint showing. Bleeding from minor lacerations can be stopped with simple measures, and does not require evacuation. Major cuts have more severe bleeding, with exposed bone, tendons, or joints. These injuries require evacuation because they require skilled surgical repair and prompt medical attention.

TREATING BLEEDING WOUNDS

1. Wash your hands with soap and water. For your own protection (and the victim's), wear clean vinyl gloves to treat all bleeding wounds. Wear sunglasses if there is a risk of blood splashing into your eye.

2. Stop all bleeding with direct finger or thumb pressure to the wound for fifteen minutes. Place rolled-up or folded sterile bandage pads or clean items of clothing (T-shirt, socks) under your fingers as pressure dressing. Note: You may need to use your entire hand for larger wounds.

3. If necessary, tie the dressing down with a strip of roller gauze or an elastic bandage. Watch for loss of pulse, coolness of skin, loss of feeling, or severe pain in any extremity beyond the pressure dressing. Loosen the dressing immediately if any of these signs or symptoms appear, but maintain pressure on the wound.

4. When the bleeding has stopped, remove the dressing and irrigate all wounds with drinkable water or sterile saline if available, using an irrigation syringe, a 30cc syringe and needle, or a large ziplock plastic bag with a small hole in it to deliver the stream of water under pressure. Clean the wound and surrounding skin with soap and water. Do not wash the wound with iodine compounds or anything else.

5. Bandage wounds after bleeding has stopped by covering them with a 3- to 4-inch sterile gauze square, wrapping lightly with roller gauze and taping. Antibiotic ointment may be applied to the sterile gauze before placing it over the wound.

6. Close any cuts that will be less painful if closed, such as those over joints, or places where the skin normally folds and creases, or those that are gaping. DO NOT close wounds with bone, tendon, or joint visible. The risk of wound infection in closed wounds is significant, and an infected wound can lead to more tissue damage than the original injury.

To close a bleeding wound safely, gently squeeze the edges of the laceration together and hold them in place with thin strips of adhesive bandage or butterfly bandages (see Fig. 17). Do not attempt to provide a watertight seal, since

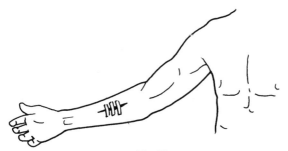

Fig. 17

some space between the strips will accommodate swelling and drainage.

8. Change the dressing immediately if it becomes soaked with blood.

9. Major lacerations associated with fractures or exposed bone, tendon, or joint should be covered (after bleeding is stopped and the wound irrigated) with sterile bandages of appropriate size, wrapped loosely with flexible gauze, and lightly taped. Such injuries require evacuation. Injuries of this kind in the lower extremities usually do not allow for self-evacuation.

Embedded Objects

All deeply embedded objects should be left in place. Never attempt to remove an embedded object. Doing so could result in severe bleeding, loss of limb, and even death. Use gauze pads placed on either side of the object to keep it from moving, and wrap with gauze rolls just as you would other wounds. Be careful not to move or compress the object further. An object embedded in the eye requires immediate medical attention (see Object in the Eye, page 169).

Wound Infection

Despite your best efforts, some wounds will get infected. An infected wound shows redness for more than a quarter inch along the margins of the wound, along with swelling, increasing pain, and possible drainage of pus. It usually takes several days to a week after the injury for an infection to become noticeable, but it can occur in as little as twenty-four hours.

TREATING INFECTED WOUNDS

1. Remove the bandage and open the wound edges by gently pulling them apart. If there is an infection the wound edges will separate easily and painlessly.

2. Irrigate the wound with water safe enough to drink; wash away all pus and tissue debris without using pressure. DO NOT use a syringe and needle to increase pressure in this case. You don't want to force infected material back into the tissue.

3. Apply antibiotic ointment lightly.

4. Re-bandage the wound with sterile bandages, leaving the wound edges apart to allow it to drain.

5. Change the bandage as often as it becomes soiled with blood or pus that soaks through; otherwise change the bandage daily.

6. If you have not done so before, start an oral antibiotic (Cephalexin is a good choice) from your first aid kit, following instructions on the label. You must be aware of medical allergies before you give anyone (including yourself) an antibiotic. Consult your physician.

9.

Blisters

Blisters have probably ruined more backcountry trips than anyone can count. A minor annoyance at home, they are potentially crippling in the backcountry if not properly cared for. Prevention of blisters is relatively simple and superior to the best treatment.

Preventing Blisters

Make sure new boots fit with the sock combination you will wear riding. Ditto with your riding apparel. Jeans or breeches should fit well without too much movement, which will reduce the amount of chafing you'll experience. Only ride in broken-in equipment. A trail ride is no time to put the miles on new gear.

On the trail, cool a "hot spot"—a painful red area that warns of blisters to come—as soon as you become aware of it. Soak the area in cold water or expose it to the air until the hot spot cools down, and change your socks or clothes for dry gear. Bandage persistent hot spots with a product such as Molefoam, 2nd Skin, or duct tape. To prevent infection, clean the area with soap and water before bandaging.

Treating Blisters

1. Clean the skin around and over the blister with mild soap. Pat dry.

2. Lightly paint the entire blister with iodine pads or solution from your first aid kit.

3. Wipe your scissors or knife with iodine, and then make a small cut in the dead skin at the bottom of the blister. This top layer of skin has already been separated from its nerve supply, so opening it should not cause pain.

4. Cover the blister area with ointment or a sterile, transparent, air- and moisture-permeable dressing; Tegaderm works well. If the area under the broken blister looks like a shallow crater or is oozing fluid or blood, cover it with a sterile hydrocolloid dressing, such as Duoderm. Blister dressings maintain a moist wound environment to promote healing, and they reduce pain.

5. Place Molefoam or a similar product over the dress-ing to pad it, and tape in place.

10.

Bone and Joint Injuries

Strains and sprains are stretching and tearing injuries to muscles, tendons, and ligaments. Along with broken bones (fractures), they are among the most common injuries. You can tell when a fracture has dislocated the parts of the bone that are broken because the injured limb looks deformed. Sometimes you can hear or feel the ends of a broken bone grating against one another. Unfortunately, not all fractures result in obvious dislocation and deformity or grating bone ends. For this reason, the initial field treatment of most sprains, strains, and fractures is similar.

Strains and Sprains

Strains and sprains are often the result of a fall. Symptoms are similar to those of a fracture, particularly in the ankle.

SIGNS OF A STRAIN OR SPRAIN

- Tenderness to the touch.

- Discoloration ("black and blue").

- Swelling in a joint or muscle.

- Pain with movement of the injured part.

TREATING STRAINS AND SPRAINS

1. A helpful memory device to recall the steps of treatment is known as RICE:

- **Rest** the injured part for forty-eight to seventy-two hours.

- **Ice** the swelling (using a plastic bag filled with ice, snow, or cold creek water). Apply cold for twenty minutes every hour, placing a towel or clean item of clothing next to the skin. Continue for forty-eight to seventy-two hours.

- **Compress** the swelling with an elastic bandage and immobilize the sprained joint.

- **Elevate** the injured part to lessen swelling and pain.

2. Treat pain with aspirin, acetaminophen, or ibuprofen.

WRAPPING AN ANKLE

In the ankle, the most commonly sprained joint, compression and splinting are accomplished with an elastic bandage by wrapping it in a cross-woven pattern.

Broken Bones

Oftentimes even a trained professional can't diagnose a broken bone without an X-ray. For first aid in the wilderness, adhere to the basic rules of splinting, immobilization, and evacuation. If displaced and dislocated fractures immediately threaten the nerve and blood supply of an extremity, the loss of blood supply below the fracture site can lead to the loss of the limb. These grossly displaced fractures must be straightened quickly if the limb is to be saved (see pages 142–143).

All fractures require evacuation and medical attention. Fractures or suspected fractures of the pelvis, hip, thigh, knee, or lower leg (tibia) require rapid evacuation to definitive treatment. Monitor for shock (see Shock, page 117).

Simple (closed) fractures are those without a break in the skin. Open fractures are fractures with any break in the skin over the fracture, up to and including those from which the ends of a bone protrude. This differentiation is important because of differences in treatment.

An adequately prepared individual must learn a great deal more about the treatment of fractures and dislocations than could be included here. Advanced splinting and immobilization techniques require professional training and practice.

SIGNS OF A SIMPLE (CLOSED) FRACTURE

- Pain and tenderness over the fracture site.

- Swelling and discoloration due to bleeding under the skin.

- Obvious deformity or severe angulation of the limb.

- The sound of bone ends grating under the skin.

- Victim cannot bear weight on injured lower extremity.

- No evidence of break in skin or protruding bone ends.

TREATING A SIMPLE FRACTURE

1. Immobilize all fractures or suspected fractures by splinting (see below). Carry a commercial flexible splint in your first aid kit or improvise with sticks, foam pads, aluminum pack stays, or rolled items of clothing and adhesive tape. DO NOT attempt to straighten a closed fracture unless it is cutting off the blood or nerve supply to the extremity, signified by numbness, tingling, extreme pain, and/or bluish color below the fracture site. Otherwise, splint it in the position in which you find it. If a fracture requires

straightening to prevent a loss of circulation in the limb, do it as soon as possible after the injury (see pages 142–143).

2. Treat swelling with ice or cold water in plastic pouches, as for a sprain.

3. Treat pain with ibuprofen according to directions on the label. (See First Aid Kit for Riders, page 173 for alternative suggestions.)

SIGNS OF AN OPEN FRACTURE

• Broken skin or visible bone ends.

• Pain and tenderness over the fracture site.

• Swelling and discoloration due to bleeding under the skin.

• Obvious deformity or severe angle of the limb.

• The sound of bone ends grating under the skin.

• Victim cannot bear weight on injured lower extremity.

TREATING AN OPEN FRACTURE

1. Irrigate the wound with water that has been made safe enough to drink until all dirt and debris are washed away. Do not close the wound with adhesive strips, staples, sutures, or glue. Instead, cover it with several bandages and tape to hold in place.

2. DO NOT attempt to straighten an open fracture unless it is cutting off the blood or nerve supply to the extremity (numbness, tingling, pain, bluish color). Otherwise splint it in the position in which you find it. If an open fracture requires straightening

to restore the blood supply or allow splinting, do it as soon as possible after the injury (see below).

3. Evacuate all open fractures as quickly as conditions allow. If evacuation is delayed more than three hours, you can administer an oral antibiotic if you have one with you. (See First Aid Kit for Riders, page 173 for suggestions.)

Straightening and Splinting

STRAIGHTENING A DEFORMED FRACTURE

Only deformed fractures that are cutting off the blood supply to an extremity should be manipulated in the field. This kind of fracture most commonly occurs in the leg, ankle, or elbow. Before you attempt fracture manipulation to save a limb that is having blood supply cut off, tell the victim what you propose to do and why, and what the risks are. The main risk is more damage to the blood supply, and more bleeding into the muscles surrounding the bone. An attempt to straighten a fracture can also fail to restore blood supply because the fractured bone ends have already cut the arterial supply. You must have the injured person's agreement and understanding before you attempt fracture manipulation.

1. One person holds the limb above the fracture site to provide an anchor for the traction. Most commonly this will be a fracture of the leg between the knee and the ankle, or the ankle, or the elbow. The person providing the anchor for the traction must not allow movement of his anchor.

2. A second person holds the extremity below the fracture site and pulls with a gentle, steady, straight pull. While maintaining gentle traction, the deformity can

be moved to normal alignment. Use the opposite, uninjured limb as a guide. The object is to restore circulation, not to provide definitive care for the fracture. Straightening the fractured bone as best you can will relieve pressure on the blood supply. If the foot or arm turns pink, warms up, and the pain is reduced, you have accomplished your goal.

3. When the fracture is straightened and circulation restored, splint to immobilize.

SPLINTING THE HAND OR FINGERS

1. Bandage the hand in a natural position with a sock or a roll of gauze in the palm (see Fig. 18).

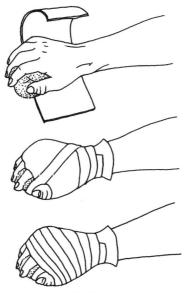

Fig. 18

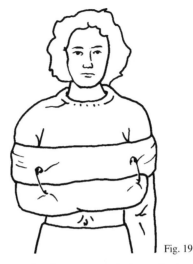

Fig. 19

2. A forearm sling is necessary to keep the hand and fingers elevated. Use a commercial triangular bandage or improvise a sling using the victim's shirt and safety pins (see Fig. 19).

SPLINTING THE WRIST OR FOREARM

1. Pad the elbow with foam from a sleeping pad or items of clothing.

2. Splint from just above elbow to palm of hand with commercial flexible splint, sticks, or whatever is handy. Wrap with elastic bandage or tape.

3. A forearm sling with an upper arm binder is necessary to keep the hand and fingers elevated and the fracture immobilized. Use a commercial triangular bandage or improvise a sling using the victim's shirt, safety pins, and an item of clothing (see Fig. 19).

SPLINTING THE ELBOW, UPPER ARM, OR SHOULDER

1. Pad the elbow with foam from a sleeping pad or items of clothing.

2. A forearm sling with an upper arm binder is necessary to keep the hand and fingers elevated and the fracture immobilized. Use a commercial triangular bandage or improvise a sling using the victim's shirt, safety pins, and an item of clothing for the binder (see Fig. 19).

3. If the fingers or hand become cool, blue, or painful, loosen the binder.

SPLINTING THE COLLARBONE

A fracture of the collarbone can be felt by running a finger over the bone. The person will report pain at the fracture site when you do this.

1. Pad under the arms to protect the nerve and blood supply.

2. Wrap an elastic bandage in a figure-8, over the clothing.

SPLINTING A FRACTURED THIGH BONE

Fractured thigh bones can cause massive internal bleeding if they are not splinted in a position of traction. For this reason, all fractured thigh bones should be splinted before evacuation. Traction is a continuous pulling force, applied temporarily by a rescuer, or longer by means of a splint. Contraction of the thigh muscles, as a reflex response to the fracture, without traction, causes severe pain. Traction

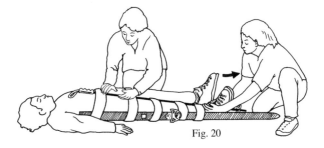

Fig. 20

makes the victim safer and far more comfortable. The splint shown in Fig. 20 and described below will provide comfort and help control bleeding around the fracture, but it is not sufficient for extended transport out of the wilderness. This injury justifies the use of helicopter evacuation.

1. One member of the party should promptly apply a gentle, straight pull (traction) from the ankle, on the ground, after the victim is evaluated. A straight pull with continuous steady force is maintained while a second member of the party prepares the splint.

2. Wrap an elastic bandage over the fracture site to control bleeding. DO NOT remove victim's boot.

3. Pad the ankle with a foam mattress cut to size, a pillow, or a jacket, and tape. Do the same around the top of the thigh where it joins the buttock.

4. Fashion a traction device (see Fig. 20,) and bandage material; duct tape works best.

5. Roll an item of clothing under the knee to flex the knee at a 5- or 10-degree position and wrap it in place with padding and tape to protect the side of the knee where the splint will be taped. A flexed knee is more comfortable during evacuation.

6. Maintain a straight, steady pull from the ankle (traction) as the splint is taped into position on the thigh and ankle padding.

7. If the foot or toes become cool, numb, or painful, loosen the ankle padding and rewrap.

8. Get help for evacuation. See pages 115–116

SPLINTING AN ANKLE, LOWER LEG, OR KNEE

1. Roll a foam pad and place it under the foot like a stirrup.

2. Wrap the padding with an elastic bandage or roller gauze and tape it in place.

3. Splints for the lower leg or knee must extend above the knee.

4. If the toe or foot becomes cool, blue, or painful, loosen the bandage.

Dislocation

A joint is dislocated when one end of a ball joint slips out of its socket, or the bones of a joint become separated. Shoulder and finger dislocations are common injuries that can be repaired by first aid methods.

Dislocations require that pain medication be given quickly and the dislocation be restored to its normal position as soon as possible. They become more difficult to treat with time due to severe muscle spasm.

SIGNS OF FINGER DISLOCATION

• Compared to other fingers, a dislocated finger looks crooked and deformed.

• Swelling and pain accompany the deformity.

TREATING A DISLOCATED FINGER

1. Grasp the base of the finger in one hand and the end of the finger in the other hand. Apply traction with a straight, steady pull until the finger appears straight when compared to the other fingers. (This will not work with the knuckle of the index finger, which requires surgery for realignment.)

2. Insert a 3- or 4-inch square cotton bandage between the fingers for padding. Splint the finger to one or two adjacent fingers with tape.

3. Medicate for pain with ibuprofen. (See First Aid Kit for Riders, page 173, for alternative medications.)

SIGNS OF DISLOCATED SHOULDER

Shoulder dislocations occur commonly in people who have had them before. They often can tell you what the diagnosis is and how to fix it.

- Shoulder loses its normal rounded shape.

- The arm is held away from the chest.

- Numbness and/or tingling in hand and arm; pulse in wrist may be weak or absent.

- Arm is weak and victim is reluctant to move it voluntarily.

TREATING A DISLOCATED SHOULDER

Treat in the field only if evacuation to medical care will require more than two hours, or if evacuation would be dangerous for the victim.

1. Have the subject lie down on a flat piece of ground. Support his arm with gentle traction as he moves into position on his back.

2. Apply a gentle, straight pull (traction) to the arm, maintaining a 90-degree angle and a bent elbow (see Fig. 21). A second person to keep the injured person from sliding is helpful.

3. Maintain a gentle, straight pull (traction) while slowly rotating the arm into a baseball pitch position (see Fig. 21).

4. Maintain position until the victim's shoulder muscles fatigue and relax, at which time the shoulder will rotate back into its socket. This can take up to fifteen minutes. Stop if pain increases. The dislocation is repaired when the pain dramatically improves and full range of movement in the arm returns.

5. Apply arm sling and binder (see Fig. 19, page 144) and evacuate to definitive medical care.

If reduction is unsuccessful, apply arm sling and binder and evacuate.

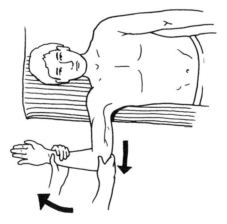

Fig. 21

11.

Lightning Injury

Although many people in the United States have experienced lightning strikes, only 20 to 30 percent of lightning strikes are fatal. Statistically, only those victims who suffer immediate cardiopulmonary arrest will die (unless they receive CPR, which is not always successful); the remainder of victims may suffer a variety of injuries, some severe, but they will survive.

It is not true that a victim of lightning strike remains "charged" and therefore a danger to her rescuers. DO NOT delay CPR in a lightning strike victim because of a fear that she will electrocute you.

Avoiding Lightning Strikes

Start rides in early morning during thunderstorm season. Plan to be back from your ride by one or two o'clock in the afternoon. Be aware of weather forecasts, and be prepared to seek shelter wherever possible.

During a thunderstorm, put down any objects with metallic components. Avoid the highest and the lowest ground. Do not seek shelter under isolated tall trees. Instead, go into thick, uniform groups of trees, brush, or boulders.

Spread your group out if caught in the open, staying ten to twenty feet apart. Maintain visual contact. Squat or crouch with your feet close together; a saddle blanket or lead rope under your feet will provide some insulation from the ground.

TREATING SOMEONE STRUCK BY LIGHTNING

Remember your ABCs—Airway, Breathing, and Circulation (see pages 110–112). And assume, for safety's sake, the victim has a neck injury until proven otherwise.

1. Stabilize the unconscious victim's head and neck before you lift the chin or move the head for your airway check and rescue breathing (see pages 110–111).

2. With the neck and spine stabilized, logroll the victim onto a sleeping pad or other insulation to keep his body off the bare ground (see Fig. 11, page 110). In wet or cold weather, cover the victim with extra clothing or sleeping bags to prevent loss of body heat.

3. Initiate CPR immediately to a breathless, pulseless victim (see CPR, pages 112–114). If the victim's heartbeat is restored, he may remain unable to breathe on his own. If this happens, continue rescue breathing during evacuation. Victims whose pulse and heartbeat do not return within thirty to forty minutes are unlikely to survive.

Survivors of lightning strike should be evacuated to definitive medical care after fractures are splinted, bleeding is controlled, and the spine immobilized (see page 128).

12.

Illness Caused by Heat

Heat edema (swelling of the hands and feet) and heat syncope (fainting, with quick recovery) are common among unacclimatized riders in hot and humid backcountry. They are not medically serious and are self-correcting, but serve as a warning to slow down, cool off, and increase fluid intake. On the other hand, heat cramps, heat exhaustion, and heat stroke are progressively severe medical conditions caused by the body's failure to adapt to hot weather. Recognition and treatment of heat cramps and heat exhaustion reduce the risk of heat stroke, a potentially fatal illness.

Obesity, poor physical conditioning, thyroid disease, diabetes, heart disease, lack of sleep, and fatigue increase your susceptibility to heat illness. Antihistamines, cold preparations, and beta-blocker blood pressure medications can interfere with sweating; if you regularly take any of these medications, consult your physician before a hot weather backcountry trip. Prevention is a whole lot easier than cure.

Preventing Heat-Related Illness

1. The most critical preventive measure is increased water intake. Don't wait until you are thirsty to replace fluids. Drink a pint (500 ml) of cool, flavored water or sport drink diluted to half strength before the start of physical activities. Drink a glassful (250 ml) every twenty to thirty minutes while exerting yourself in unaccustomed heat.

2. Maintain a pale, clear urine. Clear urine every hour or two is the goal.

3. Balanced oral replacement salts are the safest way to replace electrolyte loss during heat stress. Carry a few packages with you on trips to hot, humid climates. Avoid using salt tablets for salt replacement; they irritate the stomach and slow the entry of critical fluids into circulation.

4. Wear lightweight, light-colored, loose-fitting clothing. Lightweight cotton clothing is a good choice in hot, dry weather because it holds moisture and cools you as the moisture evaporates. In humid climates, lightweight, porous synthetics are a better choice. Avoid the windproof or waterproof versions.

5. Avoid strenuous exertion during hot, humid weather to which you are not accustomed. Start a strenuous trip at first light (or earlier) and rest in the shade during the hottest part of the day. Wait until the temperature drops late in the day to resume riding.

6. Avoid using alcohol and drugs.

Heat Cramps

Heat cramps are severe muscle cramping that begins after strenuous exercise during hot weather. Heat cramps can also be caused by consuming water with inadequate sodium replacement

TREATING HEAT CRAMPS

1. Replace lost fluids with cool water (can be flavored) to which is added a quarter teaspoon of table salt per quart (liter), or a package of balanced oral replacement solution.

2. Rest in a cool, shady spot. Resume activities when cramps are gone; gentle massage helps. If cramps return, take a rest day.

Heat Exhaustion

A more severe imbalance in the body's water and salt balance, along with an abnormal elevation of temperature (up to 104ºF), produces a more serious condition known as heat exhaustion. If you only drink when you feel thirsty, you will fall farther and farther behind in your fluid and electrolyte requirements. Untreated heat exhaustion can progress to heat stroke, a medical emergency.

You do not need a thermometer to treat heat exhaustion or heat stroke, but if you have one, so much the better. Disposable oral thermometers are available from many surgical supply distributors. They can provide a rough estimate of core temperature, which is usually about 1 degree higher than oral readings.

SIGNS OF HEAT EXHAUSTION

- Feelings of weakness, extreme fatigue, loss of appetite.

- Headaches, dizziness, sweating, rapid pulse.

- Nausea or vomiting.

- Muscle cramps.

- Skin is pale, cool, and clammy.

TREATING HEAT EXHAUSTION

1. Stop physical activities.

2. Remove victim to shade; lay the victim down with feet elevated to 30-degree angle.

3. Replace salt and water loss with cool oral rehydration solution or lightly salted water (a quarter teaspoon per quart) by mouth, at the rate of one-half glass every ten to fifteen minutes until the symptoms improve and the victim is able to produce pale to clear urine.

4. Remove hot, sweat-soaked clothing, wet the skin with cool water, and fan the victim to hasten cooling.

Recovery may take twenty-four hours. To monitor progress in heat exhaustion or heat stroke, pay close attention to the victim's improvement (or lack of improvement) in his state of alertness, level of comfort, and urine output. Fluid balance is restored when the urine is pale or colorless, and is passed two or three or more times a day. If you have a thermometer, check temperature every hour or so until it starts to drop below your first reading. If the temperature rises, increase fluid therapy until it begins to drop.

Heat Stroke

There is not always a clear line between heat exhaustion and early-stage heat stroke. The temperature of heat stroke victims is higher than that of heat exhaustion cases (105ºF or more), and heat stroke victims are less alert, more confused, and irrational. The presence of central nervous system symptoms in a heat-stressed victim is sufficient to make the field diagnosis of heat stroke.

Left untreated, heat stroke victims lapse into coma and suffer cardiac arrest. Heat stroke comes on more quickly in high-risk individuals such as children, overweight people, and the elderly, or people with heart disease, diabetes, thyroid disease, or cardiovascular disease.

SIGNS OF HEAT STROKE

- Extreme agitation, confusion, hallucinations, drowsiness, disorientation, loss of balance, or coma.

- Skin hot, dry, and red in classic cases, but some healthy young victims continue to sweat and have cool, pale skin.

TREATING HEAT STROKE

Heat stroke is life threatening. Remember your ABCs (see pages 110–112) if you are treating an unconscious victim. Start CPR if needed.

1. Cool victim as quickly as you can. Place victim in shade; lay him down with feet elevated. Remove hot, sweat-soaked clothing. Immerse victim in cold water if possible, or place plastic bags full of cold water, items of clothing soaked in cold water, or ice alongside neck, armpits, and groin, and fan the victim.

2. Do not give oral replacement fluids until victim is cooled down (temperature below 104ºF), awake, alert, and can drink without vomiting.

3. Pay close attention to improvement in the victim's state of alertness, level of comfort, ability to tolerate oral fluids, and increased urine output.

4. If you have a thermometer, check temperature every hour until it starts to drop below your first reading. If the temperature rises, increase external cooling until it begins to drop. When temperature drops below 102ºF, slow down external cooling efforts, continue oral fluids (if victim is alert enough to drink), and continue to monitor the victim.

5. Evacuate as soon as possible in all cases.

13.

Cold and Exposure Problems

Hypothermia (Low Body Temperature)

Hypothermia is defined as a drop in temperature below 95 degrees Fahrenheit. This occurs when the body loses its ability to generate enough heat to maintain normal temperature. Hypothermia claims most of its victims at environmental temperatures between 30 and 50ºF. Wind, rain, wet clothing, or falling into cold water increase the loss of heat and hasten the onset. Dehydration and inadequate calorie intake also accelerate the drop in body temperature.

You do not need to take someone's temperature in the backcountry to make the diagnosis or provide treatment. Instead, treat symptoms and monitor by paying close attention to the victim's state of alertness, level of comfort, and urine output. If your first aid kit contains a disposable oral thermometer, use the readings as a rough guide to the actual core temperature (which will usually be about 1 degree higher than the oral reading) and continue to monitor the victim for signs of improvement.

PREVENTING HYPOTHERMIA

The most important element in preventing hypothermia is to remain dry. Controlling the layer of moisture next to your skin with a layered clothing system is the most effective means of doing so.

- Lightweight or midweight synthetic tops and bottoms are a sensible first layer in any cold-weather clothing system.

- Over this layer, top and bottom, wear an ultralight nylon microfiber layer, such as a runner's windshell and windpants. This combination quickly moves moisture away from the skin. Cotton absorbs too much moisture to be effective in a cold-weather system.

- The middle layer(s) you choose depends on the air temperature, wind chill, activity level, and altitude. It should consist of a light, medium, or heavy fleece or wool top and bottom.

- Your outer layer is a windproof and waterproof shell.

In order to keep the base layer as dry as possible, adjust your pace to prevent overheating, and strip off middle layers and shell as necessary. Remember, if your hands and feet feel cold, cover your head, ears, and neck.

Other preventive steps:

- Don't wait until you are thirsty to begin to replace fluids. Drink a pint (500ml) of water before the start of a day's activities. Drink a glassful every twenty to thirty minutes while exerting yourself. Monitor the adequacy of fluid intake by maintaining a large volume of clear urine.

- Eat small snacks of nutritionally balanced food throughout the day. Carbohydrates and fats are necessary fuels for riding.

SIGNS OF MILD HYPOTHERMIA

- Person feels cold, and feet and hands may feel painfully cold.

- Shivering, the body's attempt to warm itself, begins as temperature drops below 98 to 97ºF.

- Loss of balance and coordination appears as the temperature continues to drop.

- Slurred speech is a symptom of increasingly severe hypothermia.

TREATING MILD HYPOTHERMIA

1. Find or build an emergency shelter at the onset of shivering; put up your tent, dig a snow trench, etc.

2. Build a small fire if below timberline.

3. Change into dry clothes.

4. Drink hot or warm sweet drinks. Avoid coffee or tea, since they induce excess urine output and can worsen dehydration.

5. Get into a sleeping bag, insulated from the ground. Place canteens of hot water wrapped in items of clothing inside sleeping bag, alongside your neck, groin, and armpits.

Persons who recover all faculties and normal temperature do not require evacuation.

SIGNS OF SEVERE HYPOTHERMIA

- Temperature drops below 95ºF.

- Shivering will be violent; then shivering may stop; victim can no longer rewarm herself without assistance.

- Extreme irritability and irrational judgment.

- Victim may not recognize the need to warm herself.

- Severe lack of coordination; victim may not be able to walk or stand without help.

- Level of consciousness severely impaired.

- Victim may appear to be dead (pulse, heartbeat, and breathing difficult to detect; pupils fixed and dilated), but treatment and rescue breathing should not be abandoned until the victim's body temperature is normal.

TREATING SEVERE HYPOTHERMIA

1. Move the victim to shelter gently.

2. Change her into dry clothing. Do this without sudden movements.

3. Follow all of the above measures used to field treat mild hypothermia except give nothing by mouth unless full consciousness returns. Note that rewarming may take more than a day, and may not occur at all in the field.

5. Arrange for evacuation by helicopter if possible (see Getting Help, pages 115–116).

Note: A cold or frozen person without apparent heartbeat or respiration should receive only rescue breathing; standard CPR chest compression could trigger a fatal cardiac rhythm.

Frostbite

Frostbite is a thermal injury caused by freezing of tissues. The ultimate effects of frostbite over time are similar to those of a burn of similar size and depth. Tissue is lost and function is compromised. Prevention and early recognition of frostbite are the best ways to keep fingers and toes.

PREVENTING FROSTBITE

1. Allow sufficient room in boots and gloves to avoid blood vessel constriction.

2. Wear a layered clothing system (see page 158). Do not wear cotton clothing next to your skin.

3. Maintain hydration with four to five quarts (liters) a day of clear fluid, including the water in soups and juice, in addition to snacks. This should maintain a plentiful flow of clear, colorless urine. If it does not, increase your fluid intake. In cold-weather activities, snack continuously throughout the day on nutritionally balanced foods.

4. Avoid excessive sweating; set a cold-weather pace that does not cause overheating.

SIGNS OF FROSTBITE

• Affected tissues (fingers, ears, toes, face, nose) are cold, pale, and painful.

• As depth of freezing progresses, tissue begins to turn white and feel numb. If freezing continues, tissues will become hard and stiff as ice.

TREATING FROSTBITE

1. Rewarm affected parts, immersing in water at 100 to 104ºF. Rewarm in a wilderness setting only if the following conditions are met:

a. The frostbitten extremity can be kept warm on the way out. If there is a risk it will refreeze, do not rewarm since this freeze-rewarm-freeze cycle increases tissue damage.

b. Adequate shelter and equipment (heat source, fuel, water) are available.

c. Rewarming causes considerable pain as the tissue circulation returns. Ibuprofen will control some of the pain and possibly lower the risk of tissue damage from blood clots in the injured tissue. Consult your physician. (See First Aid Kit for Riders, page 173, for alternative medications.)

2. Evacuate without rewarming if these conditions cannot be met (see Getting Help, pages 115–116).

14.

Bites and Stings

Wild Animal Bites

All victims of animal bites need to be professionally evaluated due to the risk of contracting rabies. This means you must evacuate all such victims, even those bitten by small animals or rodents. Vaccination must be accomplished as quickly as possible.

TREATING WILD ANIMAL BITES

1. Stop all bleeding. In an animal attack, there may be multiple bleeding wounds; treat as other bloody wounds (see pages 132–134). DO NOT close an animal (or human) bite wound.

2. If you are more than one day from professional medical care, start an oral antibiotic from your first aid kit following instructions on the label. You must know about medical allergies before you give anyone (including yourself) an antibiotic. Consult your physician. (See First Aid Kit for Riders, page 173, for alternative medications.)

Snakebite

According to the medical literature, a typical snakebite victim in the United States is an intoxicated, adolescent male who gets bitten while trying to handle a poisonous snake. Many, if not most, of the small number (less than ten) of snakebite deaths each year occur in this group of adolescent males when they are bitten many hours from medical care. Approximately one fourth of viper bites in North America are "dry," meaning that there is no envenomation. Most envenomations cause extreme pain at the bite site immediately, marked swelling, and severe bruising within fifteen to sixty minutes.

All accredited United States hospitals stock pit-viper antivenin. If you are generally healthy, stay calm and rational, and get to the hospital within several hours, your chances of surviving a poisonous snakebite are virtually 100 percent.

TREATING SNAKEBITES

1. Keep the victim physically and emotionally calm.

2. Clean the area gently with soap or surgical scrub.

3. Bandage lightly with a sterile bandage, 3 or 4 inches square.

4. Splint an upper extremity bite, and keep at heart level.

5. Evacuate to a medical facility without delay. Catching and killing the snake is not necessary. Current antivenin covers all North American species of pit vipers, including rattlesnakes, cottonmouths, and copperheads. Victim can walk out if able. Serious symptoms take several hours to appear.

6. DO NOT make cuts on skin or use tourniquets, pressure dressings, ice, or electrical currents to treat snakebite.

Tick Bites

Ticks are found in dry, brushy areas all over the United States; in the West they are found in sagebrush and along creek bottoms, among other places. They sense your presence by smell and jump onto you as you pass. Several illnesses are transmitted to humans by tick bites. All of them, including Lyme disease, can be cured with antibiotics if brought to a physician's attention promptly.

PREVENTING TICK BITES

During tick season (spring, summer) wear long pants and shirtsleeves. Tuck pants into socks or tape the boot-sock margin with duct tape. This prevents ticks from reaching the darker and more-difficult-to-self-examine groin, genital, and rectal areas. Wearing light-colored clothing makes it easier to find ticks that have jumped onto you.

Low-concentration DEET insect repellent (35 percent or less) can be applied to exposed skin; avoid overuse, especially in young children. (Extremely high-concentration DEET has been noted to induce cancers in mice.)

After a day outdoors in spring and summer, examine yourself and your children for ticks. Be sure to search hair, groin, and rectal areas, and look between toes and under arms. If you find a tick, don't panic. Ticks take several hours to attach themselves, and four to forty-eight hours, depending on which germs they may be carrying, to transmit disease-causing agents carried in their saliva to humans.

REMOVING A TICK

Carry a needle-nosed forceps in your first aid kit to remove the tick if it is embedded in your skin.

1. Grasp the tick close to the embedded head.

2. Pull gently in a straight back motion. Do not twist. If the entire tick is removed, a small piece of your skin will usually come off with it. Avoid crushing the

tick and contaminating your skin with tick blood and body fluids.

3. Scrub the area with soap and water or surgical scrub, and cover with a small adhesive strip bandage. Then wash your hands.

TREATING TICK BITES

If you get sick after a tick bite or develop a rash of any kind, consult your doctor. The serious illnesses caused by tick bites, including Lyme disease, can be treated successfully in the early stages—the earlier the better.

Insect Bites and Stings

Stings from bees, wasps, and yellowjackets are most common in North America. In the southeastern and parts of the southwestern United States, fire ant bites can cause a severe, life-threatening allergic reaction. About 1 percent of people are at risk for severe (anaphylactic) reaction from insect bites and stings. There are far more fatalities in the United States each year from insect stings than from snakebites.

TREATING INSECT BITES AND STINGS

1. Wash bite site with soap and water or surgical scrub.

2. Remove stinger as soon as possible if you can see it protruding from bite site. Medical research has proven that any method of removing the stinger is acceptable.

3. Apply a commercial after-bite wipe or low-concentration cortisone cream.

4. To prevent infection, cover bite with an adhesive strip bandage.

5. Use non-prescription antihistamines (such as Benadryl) to reduce itching and discomfort. (See First Aid Kit for Riders, page 173, for alternative medications.)

Severe Allergic (Anaphylactic) Reactions

Severe allergic reactions can occur as a result of many allergens including insect bites or medication allergy. Such reactions can progress to respiratory and cardiac arrest. Riders with a history of severe allergic reactions are advised to consult their physician regarding the appropriate use of an insect sting (anaphylactic) kit that contains two powerful, potentially lifesaving medications, epinephrine and diphenhydramine (often sold by the name Benadryl).

SIGNS OF SEVERE ALLERGIC (ANAPHYLACTIC) REACTION

- Rapid onset of severe itching, hives, and swelling around the bite.

- Severe swelling around lips, mouth, tongue, or throat, and difficulty swallowing.

- Rapid onset of difficulty in breathing; wheezing and chest tightness.

- Shock.

TREATING SEVERE ALLERGIC (ANAPHYLACTIC) REACTION

1. Follow the instructions on your prescription anaphylactic reaction kit (Epi-Pens come with preloaded syringes of epinephrine for self injection).

2. Be prepared to provide immediate CPR (pages 112–114).

3. Use non-prescription antihistamines (diphenhy-dramine and others) to reduce itching and swelling and to prevent recurrence of anaphylaxis symptoms.

4. Evacuate for prompt medical attention. Self-evacuation is okay if the person feels well enough to travel. Be prepared to re-administer the sting-kit medications if symptoms recur.

15.

Eye Conditions

Warning signs of a vision-threatening condition are the appearance of severe pain in the eye or diminished vision. All vision-threatening eye conditions require rapid evacuation. Self-evacuation is okay. Patch the eye for comfort (see page 170) and seek immediate medical attention.

Object in the Eye

A small foreign body may be seen easily if it is on the white part of the eye, and seen with more difficulty if lodged in the clear portion of the eye (the cornea). Use a flashlight to examine the clear part of the eye; by moving the beam of light around, you may see the foreign body. If you do not see a foreign body, retract the upper eyelid over a cotton-tipped applicator stick and look for it on the inside of the upper eyelid.

TREATING OBJECT IN THE EYE

1. Touch the tip of a moistened cotton-tipped applicator or the corner of a bandanna gently to the object. It should come away on the cotton. If it doesn't come away, irrigate the eye gently with clean water. Have the person lie down on her side, direct the stream of water into the outside corner of the eye, and allow the water to run down across the eye. Have the person blink rapidly while you do this.

2. If the object (such as a sliver of metal, rock, or fish hook) has penetrated either the white or the clear part of the eye, patch the eye and evacuate quickly to a medical facility. Self-evacuation is okay if the object is small. Pain medication may be necessary. A person with an eye patch should not travel out alone, since depth perception is impaired and the person will not be able to navigate steep or rocky trails without help.

PATCHING THE EYE

DO NOT patch red eyes that are draining a mucousy or pus-like discharge.

1. Have the person close her eye. Place several cotton balls over the lid, and place an eye patch over the cotton balls. Without cotton balls and an eye patch, a patch can be improvised by cutting soft clothing into the proper shape.

2. Secure the patch in place by taping to the forehead, the cheek, and the nose. No light should enter the patch, and the person should not require any effort to keep her eyelid closed.

16.

Water Purification

Contaminated surface water is a fact of life in the modern wilderness. Bacteria, parasites, and viruses are carried from watershed to watershed in the feces of domestic cattle, wildlife, and people. They have turned a simple drink of crystal-clear water into a risky game of chance. Three methods of disinfecting water are discussed below, and each has strengths and weaknesses. Choose a convenient primary method of disinfection depending upon your destination, equipment, and preference, and have a backup method as insurance.

Boiling

Boiling water kills all living organisms known to cause human illness. Regardless of the altitude, by the time water boils it is safe to drink; the temperature required to kill any of the organisms that cause waterborne illness, viruses included, is reached long before the boiling point. Heating water to disinfect it is virtually foolproof, but requires a stove, abundant fuel, and a pot. Pouring boiled water back and forth between containers as it cools aerates the water and improves the taste, as does mixing it with a powdered lemonade or sport drink.

Chemical Treatment

Iodine is available in several forms including Potable Aqua tablets and Polar Pure crystals. It will kill all bacteria and viruses, and all known protozoa except Cryptosporidium. In areas where Cryptosporidium is not known to exist, iodine is an excellent choice for traveling light.

However, iodine's killing power is time- and temperature-dependent. The colder and more cloudy the water, the more iodine tablets are required to disinfect it, and the longer it takes. Chlorine dioxide tablets will kill all known waterborne pathogens with a wait time of four hours. With all chemical treatments, follow the directions on the package with care.

Water Purifiers

Water filters are convenient and efficient for warm-weather trips, and most will remove parasites, cysts, and bacteria that cause human waterborne illness. On the other hand, they freeze up in cold weather, and require frequent cleaning or replacement of the filtration element. They cannot be counted on to kill all viruses that contaminate drinking water. In areas where waterborne viruses may exist, filtered water may be additionally treated with iodine.

17.

First Aid Kit for Riders

Ideally, each person or party builds or buys a first aid kit customized to suit particular needs, based on party size, length of stay in the wilderness, likelihood of professional rescue as opposed to self-rescue, pre-existing medical conditions and allergies, and the specific environmental demands of the trip. An overnight stay five miles from the trailhead in the Adirondacks of northern New York in July can present different first aid challenges than a day's ride in Idaho.

The list below is a good place to start. Larger kits and customized options are commercially available from a number of outdoor specialty shops, but resist the temptation to bring more equipment than you feel comfortable using. After you have completed courses in first aid, wilderness first response, and CPR, you will be better able to judge what kit and components are right for you.

Bandages and Surgical Supplies

- Tape, Adhesive—Use to secure splints, tape down bandages over lacerations and abrasions, etc.

- Basic Blister Dressing—Transparent, sterile film dressing such as Tegaderm for covering shallow blisters; permeable to water vapor and oxygen, impermeable to microbes.

- Spenco 2nd Skin—Hydrocolloid dressing used to cover burns; protects wound from contamination, provides rapid pain relief.

- Surgical Soap—Non-iodine, non-phenol based mild surgical soap will clean debris and contaminants from the wound surface and will not injure tissue.

- Sterile Non-Stick Bandage—4x4-inch; applied directly to cover a clean laceration or abrasion wound surface after it has been cleaned and the wound edges brought together with adhesive strips, sutured, or stapled.

- Sterile Bandage—3x3- or 4x4-inch; apply over non-adhering bandage for covering lacerations, abrasions, and open wounds; use as pressure dressing on uncontrolled bleeding of smaller wounds; use as a sterile wipe to pat dry wounds after irrigation, before dressing.

- Cotton Balls—Use for gently cleaning and wiping away dirt, grime, blood, and other secretions on skin, where sterile technique is not required.

- Iodine Wipes—Individually packaged. Use to clean skin around wound; do not apply to interior of wound.

- Vinyl Gloves—Wear these in any wound care or emergency situation where you may come into contact with bodily fluids, for protection of both the victim and yourself.

- Sterile Applicators—Useful for applying and spreading topical burn wound medication; also useful for ear wax removal, for removal of foreign body on the white part of the eye, and for examining the inside of the upper lid by gently rolling it over the stick.

- Roller Gauze—3-inch-wide, flexible, stretchy gauze; use it to wrap a wound and keep sterile pads in place. Also provides cushioning and protection for the injury.

- Adhesive Plastic Bandage Strips—1-inch wide; for covering minor cuts, scrapes, insect bites, and blisters.

- Sunscreen—SPF 15 at least; more at high altitude.

- Insect Sting Stick or Wipes—Apply to insect bites or stings for relief of discomfort.

- Flexible Splinting (SAM splint™)—Moldable aluminum splint covered with closed cell foam, marketed under the trade name SAM splint™. Can be cut to size and shape as needed for use on wrist, arm, elbow, or ankle.

- Wound Closure Strips—Use to bring together the skin edges of minor cuts.

- Eye Pads—To cover an injured, painful, sunblind, or red eye to provide comfort and protection.

- Tongue Depressors—Use to examine a mouth, throat, or tongue condition, or as small splints for finger injuries; also useful for applying ointments to a large area or as tinder for an emergency fire.

- Molefoam—Pressure point padding, often used in conjunction with adhesive or duct tape to prevent blisters in known pressure points. Molefoam is a padded (and thus more comfortable) version of another blister-preventative product called Moleskin.

- Duct Tape—Use for fashioning splints, preventing hot spots on feet, immobilizing the neck and spine, and other uses.

- Cyanoacrylate Glue (SuperGlue)—Use for closing those small, clean, but hard-to-bandage nicks, scrapes, and cuts on fingers, knuckles, and hands that seem to stay open forever.

Specialized Medical Instruments

- Wound Irrigation Syringe—To provide adequate pressure for washing dirt, debris, and microbes from the wound.

- Anaphylaxis Emergency Kit—Commercially available by prescription only; follow the instructions on the kit exactly.

- Forceps—4.5-inch; use for removing foreign bodies such as splinters, bee stingers, cactus spines, etc.

- Scissors—4.5-inch; use to trim or cut off bandages, splints, or hair around a scalp wound before treatment.

- Airway Kit—Assorted sizes, child and adult; use to maintain an open upper airway when you perform CPR or rescue breathing.

- Survival ("Space") Blanket—Thin, extremely lightweight reflective blanket used to conserve body heat.

Non-Prescription Medications

- Hydrocortisone Cream—1 percent strength; apply a small amount to insect bites, stings, poison ivy, or poison oak skin rashes three or four times a day.

- Decongestant Nasal Spray—For colds, stuffy nose, and blocked sinuses of any cause.

- Bismuth Salicylate Tablets (Pepto-Bismol)—Antidiarrheal, anti-indigestion medication.

- Diphenhydramine—25 mg tablets; antihistamine for symptoms of allergy; also used as sleep medication.

- Pain Medication—Aspirin, acetaminophen (Tylenol), and ibuprofen each provide varying amounts of pain relief depending on individual responses.

Prescription Medications
(Consult Your Physician)

- Lorazepam 0.5 mg—A sedative useful for treating acute stress reactions. Can be habit forming. Not for use at high altitude because it slows respiration.

- Pain Medication: Acetaminophen (Tylenol) with Codeine—Oral pain relief equivalent to injectable morphine, with the same risks: depressed respiration at high altitude, daytime drowsiness, nausea, or vomiting. Can be habit forming.

- Oral Antibiotic: Cephalexin (Keflex)—Used to treat skin and wound infections, and for open fractures if evacuation is delayed.

- Oral Antibiotic: Trimethoprim/Sulfamethoxazole— Useful for treatment of upper respiratory infection, bladder or urinary tract infection, and as an alternative treatment for traveler's diarrhea.

- Oral Antibiotic: Erythromycin (various forms)—Used in place of penicillin or Cephalexin in penicillin-allergic people.

Acknowledgments

I would like to thank Mark Borke, MD, emergency medicine specialist in Butte, Montana, and John Bleicher, teacher and education coordinator of Missoula EMS, for their professional wisdom and contributions in the review of the medical material in this book. For those readers who would like to learn as much as they can about the challenging area of emergency wilderness medicine, John's five-day course in Wilderness First Response, given in Missoula, Montana, every winter, is one of the very best anywhere.

Jim Wilson, a dedicated mountaineer and veteran of numerous Alaskan expeditions, among other climbing accomplishments, deserves many thanks for invaluable suggestions offered from a true wilderness expert's point of view.

Special thanks go to Bill Schneider, Falcon publisher, for providing me the opportunity to write this book, and to Russ Schneider, editor and veteran Glacier Wilderness Guide.

—Gilbert Preston

Index

Italicized page numbers indicate illustrations.

About the Authors

Nancy S. Loving, DVM, has been both a dressage and event competitor and has been involved in the endurance world as an FEI–sanctioned veterinarian and as team vet for the USEF national endurance squad. Prior to becoming an avid endurance rider training her horses in the National Forest outside her back door, Dr. Loving spent two months horse camping across the wilderness backcountry of Colorado. Dr. Loving graduated from Colorado State University Veterinary School in 1985, and since then has practiced equine medicine and surgery exclusively. She regularly writes for *The Horse* and *Horse Illustrated* magazines, and her previous books include *All Horse Systems Go: The Horse Owner's Full-Color Veterinary Care and Conditioning Resource for Modern Performance, Sport and Pleasure Horses; Go the Distance: The Complete Resource for Endurance Horses; Conformation and Performance;* and *Veterinary Manual for the Performance Horse.*

Gilbert Preston, MD, has practiced primary care medicine in rural Montana for more than twenty years. A former research associate at the National Institutes of Health in Bethesda, Maryland, Dr. Preston is a member of the Wilderness Medical Society and is currently on staff at Saint James Community Hospital in Butte, Montana. He has published more than two hundred medical articles in Pacific Northwest newspapers and magazines.

Dr. Preston is also the founder and medical director of Wilderness Medical Systems in Butte, Montana.